WOMAN'S HORMONE HANDBOOK

WOMAN'S HORMONE HANDBOOK

UNLOCK THE SECRETS OF FEMALE HORMONAL
HEALTH FOR LIFELONG BALANCE AND VITALITY

WOMEN'S HEALTH

LILA LACY

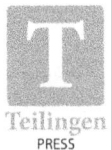

Copyright © 2024 by Lila Lacy

All rights reserved. No part of this book may be reproduced, stored in a retrieval system, or transmitted in any form or by any means, electronic, mechanical, photocopying, recording, or otherwise, without the prior written permission of the publisher, Teilingen Press.

The information contained in this book is based on the author's personal experiences and research. While every effort has been made to ensure the accuracy of the information presented, the author and publisher cannot be held responsible for any errors or omissions.

This book is intended for general informational purposes only and is not a substitute for professional medical, legal, or financial advice. If you have specific questions about any medical, legal, or financial matters matters, you should consult with a qualified healthcare professional, attorney, or financial advisor.

Teilingen Press is not affiliated with any product or vendor mentioned in this book. The views expressed in this book are those of the author and do not necessarily reflect the views of Teilingen Press.

To all the women who seek harmony within,
May this book light your path to understanding and wellness.

For the mothers, daughters, sisters, and friends—
Your health is your story; let this be a guiding pen.

Balance is not something you find, it's something you create.

— JANA KINGSFORD

CONTENTS

Embracing Hormonal Harmony — xi

1. UNDERSTANDING HORMONES: THE BASICS — 1
   The Endocrine System: A Symphony of Glands — 3
   Hormones and Women: A Unique Relationship — 4
   The Lifecycle of Female Hormones — 6
   Common Hormonal Disorders in Women — 7
   Chapter Summary — 9

2. PUBERTY TO FERTILITY: THE REPRODUCTIVE YEARS — 11
   The Menstrual Cycle: A Monthly Rhythm — 13
   Understanding Ovulation and Fertility — 14
   Contraception and Hormonal Control — 16
   Polycystic Ovary Syndrome: Insights and Management — 17
   Chapter Summary — 19

3. PREGNANCY AND HORMONES: THE MIRACLE OF LIFE — 21
   The Role of Hormones in Fetal Development — 23
   Managing Hormonal Fluctuations in Pregnancy — 24
   Postpartum Hormonal Adjustments — 26
   Breastfeeding and Hormonal Effects — 27
   Chapter Summary — 29

4. PERIMENOPAUSE AND MENOPAUSE: TRANSITIONING PHASES — 31
   Understanding Menopause: Symptoms and Signs — 33
   Hormone Replacement Therapy: Pros and Cons — 35
   Natural Approaches to Menopausal Symptoms — 36
   Bone Health and Hormones in Aging Women — 38
   Chapter Summary — 40

5. THYROID HEALTH: THE METABOLIC REGULATOR — 43
   Hypothyroidism: When the Thyroid Slows Down — 45
   Hyperthyroidism: The Overactive Thyroid — 46
   Autoimmune Thyroid Diseases: Hashimoto's and Graves' — 48

Nutrition and Lifestyle for Thyroid Health	49
Chapter Summary	51

6. STRESS AND HORMONES: THE ADRENAL CONNECTION — 53
Cortisol: The Stress Hormone — 54
Adrenal Fatigue: Myth or Reality? — 56
Strategies for Managing Stress and Hormonal Balance — 57
Stress and Female Hormonal Disorders — 59
Chapter Summary — 61

7. WEIGHT, METABOLISM, AND HORMONES — 63
Insulin Resistance and Its Impact on Health — 65
Leptin and Ghrelin: Hunger Hormones Explained — 66
The Thyroid-Weight Connection — 68
Hormonal Strategies for Weight Management — 69
Chapter Summary — 71

8. MOOD, BRAIN FUNCTION, AND HORMONES — 73
Estrogen and Cognitive Function — 75
The Serotonin Connection and PMS — 76
Hormones and Mental Health Disorders — 78
Lifestyle Choices for Hormonal Mood Regulation — 79
Chapter Summary — 81

9. SKIN, HAIR, AND HORMONES — 83
Acne and Hormones: Beyond the Teenage Years — 84
Hair Loss and Excess Hair Growth: Hormonal Influences — 86
Natural Approaches to Hormonal Skin and Hair Health — 87
The Impact of Diet on Skin and Hair — 89
Chapter Summary — 91

10. INTEGRATIVE APPROACHES TO HORMONE HEALTH — 93
The Role of Diet in Hormone Balance — 94
Exercise and Hormonal Health — 95
Sleep's Influence on Hormonal Regulation — 97
Mind-Body Practices for Hormonal Harmony — 98
Navigating Hormone Therapy and Supplements — 100
Chapter Summary — 102

Your Hormonal Journey — 103

About the Author — 109

EMBRACING HORMONAL HARMONY

Welcome to the intricate world of hormones, the unsung heroes orchestrating the vast symphony of womanhood. These potent chemical messengers are pivotal in every chapter of a woman's life, from the awakening of puberty to the transformative waves of menopause.

Every day and night, your hormones work harmoniously to create the rich and dynamic experience of being a woman. Hormones like estrogen and progesterone ebb and flow, shaping reproductive health and influencing everything from your mood to your metabolism.

The "Woman's Hormone Handbook" is designed to illuminate these complex interactions, providing you with the knowledge to understand your body's signals and act upon them. In this book, we'll embark on an enlightening journey to decode the whispers and roars of your hormonal landscape. Understanding these signals is crucial, as they influence not just physical health but also emotional well-being and mental clarity. As we unfold the pages of this guide, you'll gain insights into how to harmonize your body's natural rhythms, empowering you to live with vitality and grace.

You'll discover how to listen to your body's hormonal cues and respond with informed, nurturing choices. Whether navigating the tides of fertility or seeking solace in the flux of hormonal shifts, this book is your compass to a balanced and vibrant existence. It is more than a guide; it celebrates the female body's innate wisdom. Together, we'll explore the beauty and challenges of each hormonal shift, equipping you with the tools to thrive through every phase of life.

The Endocrine System

Imagine the endocrine system as a magnificent orchestra, with each gland playing a vital role in the symphony of your body's functions. This complex network of glands and hormones works in unison to regulate everything from growth and metabolism to mood and reproduction. We'll delve into the intricacies of this system, demystifying how it conducts the rhythms of daily life, and you'll learn how each gland and hormone can affect your well-being. Disruptions in this delicate balance may lead to conditions such as thyroid disorders or adrenal fatigue, which can profoundly impact your quality of life.

Understanding the endocrine system's melody is essential to mastering your hormonal health. With the knowledge you'll gain from these pages, you'll be equipped to fine-tune your body's hormonal orchestra, ensuring that each gland plays its part beautifully and you experience the full, rich symphony of optimal health.

Hormonal Challenges and Triumphs

Navigating the ebb and flow of hormones is a central part of life. In this book, we'll also explore the common hormonal challenges many women encounter, acknowledging the struggles and celebrating the triumphs that come with each. Conditions like Polycystic Ovary Syndrome and thyroid imbalances are more than mere inconveniences; they are puzzles that, when solved, can unlock a new level of wellness and self-understanding.

You'll find empowering strategies to manage and mitigate their effects, turning a challenge into a victory for your health. We'll explore how to confidently navigate their symptoms, using both time-tested remedies and modern medical advancements.

A Holistic Approach to Hormone Health

This book doesn't shy away from the role of medical interventions, including hormone replacement therapy and supplements. Instead, it places these within a larger context of self-care and informed choice. Hormonal health is not merely the absence of disease; it's a state of complete harmony where lifestyle, nutrition, and medical care converge. By embracing a holistic approach, you'll learn to navigate the nuances of your hormonal health, crafting a personalized plan that resonates with your body's needs and your life's unique demands.

Your Companion on the Journey to Well-being

The "Woman's Hormone Handbook" is your guide to a more vibrant, balanced you. It is more than a mere collection of facts and advice; it is a steadfast companion on your personal journey to well-being. As you turn each page, you'll find a supportive guide that understands the intricacies of your body's hormonal ebb and flow. This book is a testament to the belief that knowledge is power—the power to heal, balance, and thrive.

Embarking on this journey, you'll be equipped with a deep understanding of how hormones impact every facet of your health. From the physical changes of puberty to the emotional swings of menopause, this handbook provides clarity and comfort. It's a resource you can return to time and again, finding answers to your questions and solace in shared experiences.

The journey to hormonal well-being is not a straight path—it's a winding road filled with discoveries and learning opportunities. As your companion, this book offers easy to understand explanations and practical, real-world applications. It empowers you to make informed decisions about your health, whether you're considering dietary changes, lifestyle adjustments, or medical treatments.

Embracing Hormonal Harmony

Above all, this book celebrates womanhood in all its complexity. It encourages you to embrace your body's signals, listen intently, and respond with love and care. Your journey to hormonal harmony is a profound one, and with this book in hand, you're never alone. Together, we'll navigate the path to a balanced and fulfilling life where well-being is your destination. So, are you ready to begin?

1
UNDERSTANDING HORMONES: THE BASICS

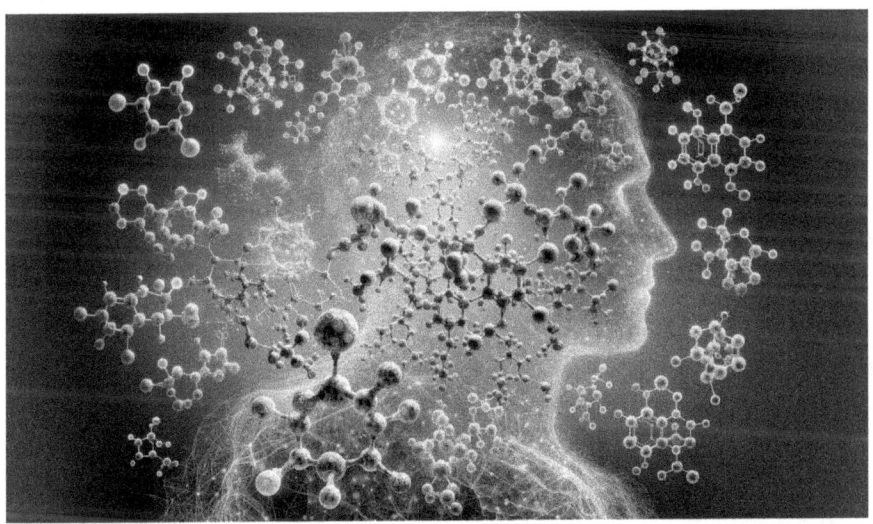

Imagine your body as a complex network, a bustling city where communication is vital to maintaining order and balance. In this city, hormones are the messengers, the whispers and shouts that travel through the bloodstream, carrying vital information from one part of the body to another. They are the chemical signals that orchestrate many bodily functions, from growth and metabolism to mood and reproduction.

Hormones are produced by various glands and organs within the body, each with a specific set of responsibilities. These glands are like unique broadcasting stations, sending messages to target cells equipped with the right receivers – hormone receptors. When a hormone docks onto its receptor, it delivers its message, prompting the cell to perform a particular action or initiate a series of events.

The beauty of hormones lies in their diversity and specificity. Some, like insulin, regulate the sugar level in our blood, ensuring that our cells receive the energy they need. Others, such as estrogen and progesterone, play pivotal roles in the reproductive system, influencing menstrual cycles, pregnancy, and even the health of our bones and heart.

But hormones are not solo artists; they perform in a finely-tuned ensemble. The balance between different hormones is crucial. Too much or too little of a single hormone can disrupt this balance, leading to a variety of health issues. For women, this balance is particularly delicate, as their bodies undergo significant hormonal changes throughout life – from the onset of puberty to the transition of menopause.

Understanding hormones is akin to learning a new language, one that can explain why we feel the way we do, why our bodies change over time, and how we can better support our health by listening to the subtle yet powerful signals they send us. As we delve deeper into the world of hormones, we'll discover how this intricate system of chemical messengers influences our physical well-being, emotions, and behaviors.

So, let's continue our journey into the next section, where we'll explore the endocrine system – the network of glands that compose the grand symphony of hormone production and regulation in our bodies. By understanding this system, we'll gain insights into how to maintain harmony within, ensuring that each gland plays its part beautifully in the concert of our health.

The Endocrine System: A Symphony of Glands

Imagine an orchestra, each musician poised with an instrument, ready to play their part in a complex musical piece. This is akin to the endocrine system in our bodies—a collection of glands that work in concert to produce and release hormones, the body's chemical messengers. Each gland in the endocrine system has a specific role, much like each musician in an orchestra has a particular part to play. Together, they create a harmony that regulates various bodily functions, from growth and metabolism to reproduction and mood.

The maestro of this symphony is the hypothalamus, a small but mighty region of the brain. It's the conductor, directing the pituitary gland, often called the 'master gland,' through signals that determine the release of hormones. The pituitary gland, in response, sends its own signals to other glands in the body, such as the thyroid, adrenals, and the reproductive organs—the ovaries in women.

The thyroid gland, nestled in the front of your neck, plays the notes that regulate your metabolism, energy levels, and even how warm you feel. It's like the orchestra's string section, setting the pace and tone for many bodily functions.

The adrenal glands, perched atop your kidneys like tiny hats, produce hormones like cortisol and adrenaline. These are the brass instruments that sound the alarm and energize the body in times of stress or excitement.

For women, the ovaries are the soloists of the hormone symphony, producing estrogen and progesterone. These hormones are central to reproductive health, influencing menstrual cycles, pregnancy, and even the transition into menopause.

Each gland works in response to the others, with feedback loops fine-tuning the performance. Suppose one musician plays too loudly or softly or misses a cue. In that case, the harmony is disrupted, leading to various health issues. For example, an overactive thyroid can cause symptoms like anxiety and weight loss. In contrast, an underactive thyroid might lead to fatigue and weight gain.

Maintaining this delicate balance is crucial for overall health, and it's especially important for women, whose hormonal needs change throughout their lives. Understanding how these glands work together helps us appreciate the complexity and beauty of our bodies. It underscores the importance of taking care of our hormonal health.

As we move forward, we'll explore the unique relationship women have with their hormones and how this connection influences their health at every stage of life. Just as every note in a symphony is essential to the beauty of the whole piece, every hormone in your body plays a vital role in your overall well-being.

Hormones and Women: A Unique Relationship

In the intricate dance of the endocrine system, women's bodies play a particularly complex tune. Hormones, those chemical messengers that traverse our bloodstream to regulate physiology and behavior, profoundly impact women's health. Their influence begins at puberty and wends its way through the phases of adulthood, from the potential for pregnancy to the transition of menopause.

For women, hormones do more than just regulate the reproductive system. They are pivotal in determining many bodily functions, including but not limited to metabolism, bone density, and even mood. Estrogen and progesterone, the primary female sex hormones, are often the stars of the show. They're supported by a cast of others like testosterone, which women produce in smaller amounts, and thyroid hormones, cortisol, and insulin.

The relationship between women and their hormones is unique, not only because of the cyclical nature of the female reproductive system but also because of how these hormones interact with each other and different body systems. For instance, estrogen plays a crucial role in maintaining healthy bones, and a drop in its levels during menopause can lead to an increased risk of osteoporosis. Similarly, hormonal fluctuations can affect mental health, with some women experiencing mood swings, anxiety, or depression as hormone levels ebb and flow during the menstrual cycle, pregnancy, or menopause.

Understanding this relationship is crucial because it underscores the importance of hormone balance in overall health. When hormones are in harmony, they facilitate the smooth operation of bodily functions. However, when imbalances occur, they can lead to a range of health issues, from menstrual irregularities and skin problems to more serious conditions like polycystic ovary syndrome (PCOS) or thyroid disorders.

Moreover, the influence of hormones extends beyond physical health. They can affect emotional well-being, influencing how you feel and perceive the world around you. It's not uncommon for women to notice changes in their emotional state at different points in their menstrual cycle, and these shifts are a testament to the powerful effects hormones have on the brain and nervous system.

It's also important to recognize that everyone's hormonal journey is unique. Factors such as genetics, lifestyle, stress levels, and environmental exposures can all influence hormone health. This means that while there are general patterns and shared experiences, each woman's hormonal profile and how it affects her health and well-being is highly individual.

By embracing a holistic view of hormone health, you can better understand your body and take proactive steps toward maintaining hormonal balance. This might include lifestyle changes such as diet and exercise, stress management techniques, or, when necessary, seeking medical advice and treatment options.

In the next part of our exploration, we will delve into the lifecycle of female hormones, tracing their ebbs and flows from the onset of menstruation to menopause. This journey will illuminate not only the biological milestones of a woman's life but also how these hormonal shifts can be navigated to maintain health and vitality at every stage.

The Lifecycle of Female Hormones

As we delve into the intricate world of female hormones, we must recognize that their journey is not static. The lifecycle of female hormones is a dynamic and continuous process, evolving from puberty through menopause. This journey is marked by a symphony of hormonal fluctuations that influence reproductive health and play a significant role in overall well-being.

Let's begin with puberty, a time of significant change as the body transitions from childhood into reproductive maturity. This period is characterized by the activation of the hypothalamic-pituitary-gonadal axis, which orchestrates the production and regulation of critical hormones like estrogen and progesterone. These hormones are responsible for the development of secondary sexual characteristics and the initiation of menstrual cycles.

As a young woman's body adapts to these changes, the menstrual cycle becomes a central aspect of hormonal health. Each cycle can be divided into distinct phases: the follicular phase, ovulation, and the luteal phase. During the follicular phase, the hormone estrogen rises, leading to the maturation of an ovarian follicle. Ovulation then marks the release of an egg. This moment hinges on a delicate balance of luteinizing hormone (LH) and follicle-stimulating hormone (FSH). Following ovulation, the luteal phase increases progesterone, preparing the uterine lining for potential pregnancy.

If pregnancy does not occur, the cycle concludes with menstruation, and the hormonal dance begins anew. It's important to acknowledge that while this cycle is described in a neat sequence, many women experience variations in cycle length and hormone levels, which are entirely normal.

As women age, they eventually encounter perimenopause, the transitional period leading up to menopause. This stage can last several years and is marked by more pronounced hormonal fluctuations. Estrogen and progesterone levels may rise and fall unpredictably, leading to changes in menstrual patterns and, often, the onset of symptoms such as hot flashes, night sweats, and mood swings.

Finally, menopause is reached when a woman has not menstruated for 12 consecutive months. At this point, the ovaries have ceased releasing eggs and producing most of their estrogen. While menopause is a natural biological process, the decline in estrogen can have widespread effects on the body, including changes in bone density, cardiovascular health, and skin elasticity.

Throughout each of these stages, it's crucial to understand that hormone levels are not just reproductive signals; they influence a myriad of systems in the body. From emotional regulation to metabolic processes, hormones are integral to maintaining balance and health.

As we move forward, we will explore how disruptions in this delicate hormonal balance can lead to various disorders. By understanding the typical lifecycle of female hormones, we can better recognize when something may be amiss and take steps to address these issues with compassion and knowledge.

Common Hormonal Disorders in Women

As we delve deeper into the intricacies of hormone health, it's essential to understand that the delicate balance of hormones can sometimes be disrupted, leading to various disorders that can significantly impact a woman's quality of life. These disorders can manifest at any stage, from the onset of puberty to post-menopause, and understanding them is the first step towards managing and treating them effectively.

One of the most common hormonal disorders affecting women is Polycystic Ovary Syndrome (PCOS). This condition is characterized by an imbalance of reproductive hormones, which can lead to a variety of symptoms, including irregular menstrual cycles, acne, excessive hair growth, and difficulties with fertility. Women with PCOS may also experience insulin resistance, which can increase the risk of developing type 2 diabetes.

Another disorder that is frequently encountered is thyroid dysfunction, which can come in the form of hypothyroidism or hyperthyroidism. The thyroid gland plays a crucial role in regulating metabolism, and any imbalance can lead to symptoms such as weight gain or loss, fatigue, changes in heart rate, and mood disturbances. Hypothyroidism, where the thyroid produces insufficient hormones, is more common and can be particularly challenging for women, as it can also affect menstrual regularity and fertility.

Menstrual disorders such as premenstrual syndrome (PMS) and premenstrual dysphoric disorder (PMDD) also have a hormonal basis. While PMS is relatively common, and its symptoms—such as bloating, mood swings, and breast tenderness—are familiar to many, PMDD is a more severe form that can be debilitating. PMDD can cause extreme mood shifts and has a profound impact on a woman's emotional and physical well-being.

During the transition to menopause, known as perimenopause, women may experience hormonal fluctuations that can lead to symptoms like hot flashes, night sweats, sleep disturbances, and mood swings. This period can last several years and is a natural part of aging. Still, for some women, the symptoms can be severe enough to disrupt daily life.

Endometriosis is another condition that, while not solely a hormonal disorder, is influenced by hormonal activity. This painful condition occurs when tissue similar to the lining of the uterus grows outside of it, leading to severe pain, irregular bleeding, and potential fertility issues. Hormones play a role in the growth of this tissue, and managing hormonal levels can be a crucial aspect of treatment.

Lastly, hormonal imbalances can also lead to conditions such as osteoporosis, particularly after menopause, when the protective effects of estrogen decline. This can result in a decrease in bone density, making bones more fragile and susceptible to fractures.

Hormones are powerful messengers in our bodies. When their messages go awry, the effects can be far-reaching. However, many of these disorders can be treated effectively with proper diagnosis and management. It's essential to be attuned to your body and seek medical advice when you notice changes that could indicate a hormonal imbalance. By doing so, you can take proactive steps toward maintaining your hormonal health and overall well-being.

Chapter Summary

- Hormones are chemical messengers that regulate bodily functions, including growth, metabolism, mood, and reproduction. They are produced by various glands and organs.
- The balance of hormones is crucial for health, with imbalances causing issues; women's hormonal balance is particularly delicate due to life changes like puberty and menopause.
- The endocrine system consists of glands that produce hormones, with the hypothalamus and pituitary glands directing other glands like the thyroid and adrenals.
- Women have a unique relationship with hormones, affecting not just reproduction but also metabolism, bone density, and mood, with estrogen and progesterone playing central roles.
- Hormonal imbalances in women can lead to health issues like menstrual irregularities, PCOS, and thyroid disorders and also affect emotional well-being.
- The lifecycle of female hormones involves puberty, menstrual cycles, perimenopause, and menopause, impacting reproductive health and overall well-being.
- Common hormonal disorders in women include PCOS, thyroid dysfunction, menstrual disorders like PMS and PMDD, perimenopausal symptoms, endometriosis, and osteoporosis post-menopause.
- Understanding and managing hormonal health is crucial for women, with lifestyle changes and medical treatment helping to maintain balance and address disorders.

2
PUBERTY TO FERTILITY: THE REPRODUCTIVE YEARS

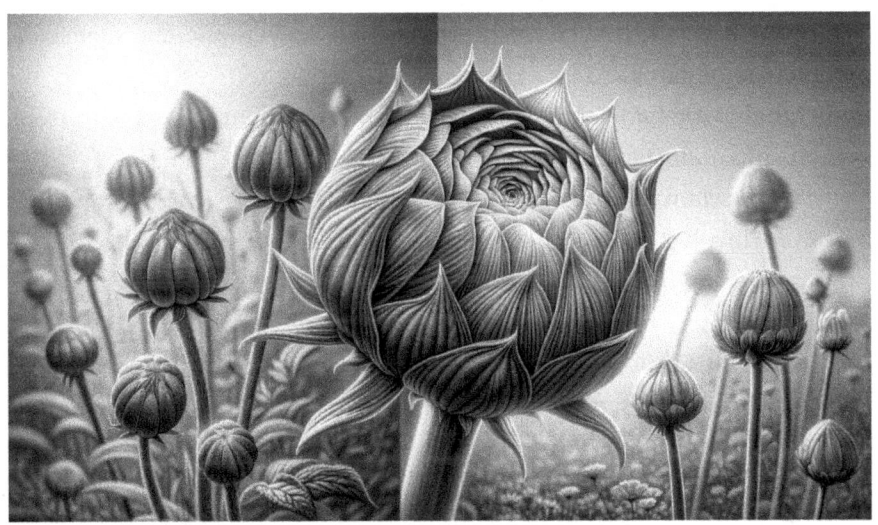

As the first whispers of womanhood begin, puberty ushers in a symphony of hormonal changes that transform the female body. This period of life is marked by the onset of menstruation, a milestone in reproductive maturity. It is the culmination of intricate hormonal events that deserve our understanding and respect.

The hormonal awakening typically begins between the ages of 8 and 13, when the hypothalamus, a master gland in the brain, releases gonadotropin-releasing hormone (GnRH). This hormone signals the pituitary gland to produce two other key players in the reproductive symphony: follicle-stimulating hormone (FSH) and luteinizing hormone (LH). These hormones travel through the bloodstream to the ovaries, which house thousands of dormant eggs.

In response to FSH and LH, the ovaries mature some of these eggs and produce the hormones estrogen and progesterone. Estrogen mainly plays a pivotal role in the development of secondary sexual characteristics, such as the growth of breasts, the widening of hips, and the appearance of pubic and underarm hair. It also contributes to the growth spurt that often accompanies puberty.

As estrogen levels rise, it triggers the thickening of the lining of the uterus, preparing it for the potential of pregnancy. If fertilization does not occur, the body must shed this lining, which leads to the first menstrual period, or menarche. The experience of menarche is as unique as the individual, with some girls greeting it with excitement, others with trepidation, and many with a mix of emotions.

It's important to note that the first few cycles can be irregular and may not even involve ovulation. This irregularity is expected as the body is still fine-tuning its hormonal communication. Over time, cycles generally settle into a more predictable pattern.

During this time, it is not uncommon for young women to experience a range of symptoms, from mood swings to cramps, as their bodies adjust to the ebb and flow of hormones. These experiences, while sometimes uncomfortable or confusing, are a normal part of the journey toward reproductive maturity.

As we embrace this hormonal awakening, providing support and education is crucial. Understanding the changes can empower young women to take charge of their health and well-being. Open conversations about menstruation, mood changes, and the physical transformations of puberty can demystify this natural process and foster a positive body image.

Remember, puberty is not just a biological event; it's a transition into a new phase of life with its own challenges and triumphs. As we move forward, we'll explore how the monthly rhythm of the menstrual cycle becomes a central part of a woman's life, influencing her health and well-being in profound ways.

The Menstrual Cycle: A Monthly Rhythm

As we journey through the reproductive years, the menstrual cycle is a testament to the intricate dance of hormones within a woman's body. This cycle, typically lasting around 28 days, though it can range from 21 to 35 days, is not just a biological process but a barometer of health and well-being.

At the heart of the menstrual cycle is the ebb and flow of hormones, primarily estrogen and progesterone, produced by the ovaries. These hormones work in a delicate balance, orchestrating the preparation of the uterus for potential pregnancy and the release of an egg during ovulation.

The cycle begins on the first day of menstruation, a phase commonly known as the period. This is when the lining of the uterus, which had thickened in preparation for a fertilized egg, is shed because pregnancy has not occurred. Menstruation can last anywhere from 2 to 7 days. While symptoms like cramping and mood swings can accompany it, it's a natural part of the cycle.

Following menstruation, the body enters the follicular phase. During this time, the pituitary gland releases follicle-stimulating hormone (FSH), which encourages the growth of ovarian follicles, each containing an immature egg. One of these follicles will become dominant and mature while the body reabsorbs the others.

As the dominant follicle grows, it produces more estrogen, which signals the lining of the uterus to thicken again, creating a nurturing environment for a potential embryo. This rise in estrogen also triggers a surge in luteinizing hormone (LH), which leads to the next pivotal event: ovulation.

Ovulation is the release of the mature egg from the ovary into the fallopian tube, where it awaits fertilization. This fertility window is narrow, with the egg remaining viable for about 24 hours. If sperm are present during this time, conception may occur.

Should fertilization not take place, the cycle progresses to the luteal phase. The ruptured follicle transforms into the corpus luteum, which secretes progesterone. Progesterone maintains the uterine lining, but without a pregnancy, its levels will eventually fall, leading to the shedding of the lining and the start of a new menstrual period.

Throughout these phases, women may experience a variety of symptoms, from the bloating and mood changes of premenstrual syndrome (PMS) to the heightened senses and energy around ovulation. It's important to remember that each woman's experience of her menstrual cycle is unique, and variations in cycle length, symptoms, and flow are all part of the spectrum of normal.

Understanding the menstrual cycle is more than just a matter of biology; it's about tuning into the rhythms of one's own body. By recognizing the patterns and signals of their cycles, women can gain insights into their overall health, plan for or prevent pregnancy, and make informed decisions about their reproductive health.

As we move forward, we'll delve deeper into the specifics of ovulation and fertility, unraveling the signs and processes crucial to conception and the continuation of these reproductive years.

Understanding Ovulation and Fertility

As we journey through the reproductive years, a fundamental aspect to grasp is the process of ovulation and its pivotal role in fertility. Ovulation is the release of an egg from one of the ovaries. This moment is both fleeting and fertile, marking a window of opportunity for conception.

Each month, in response to a symphony of hormonal signals, a select group of eggs, or oocytes, begin to mature within the ovarian follicles. Typically, one egg outpaces the others and reaches full maturity. This surge is orchestrated by a rise in follicle-stimulating hormone (FSH), which nudges the follicles into action, and luteinizing hormone (LH), which peaks just before ovulation, triggering the release of the egg.

The journey of the egg is a delicate voyage. Once released, it is swept into the fallopian tube, where it may meet sperm and become fertilized. This is where timing becomes crucial. The egg remains viable for about 12 to 24 hours post-ovulation, while sperm can survive in the female reproductive tract for up to five days. Therefore, the days leading up to and including ovulation constitute the fertile window.

Understanding one's fertility can be empowering. Many women learn to recognize the signs of ovulation, such as a change in cervical mucus, which becomes more transparent and more stretchy, akin to egg whites, and a slight rise in basal body temperature following ovulation. Others may experience ovulation pain, known as mittelschmerz, a dull ache, or a sharp twinge on one side of the lower abdomen.

Tracking these signs can be incredibly helpful for those trying to conceive, as it helps pinpoint the most fertile days. However, it's important to remember that each woman's cycle is unique, and these signs can vary widely. For some, ovulation can occur like clockwork, while for others, it may be more unpredictable.

For women not looking to conceive, understanding ovulation is equally essential. It informs choices around contraception and can shed light on various health conditions that may affect or be affected by the menstrual cycle. Moreover, it fosters a deeper connection with one's body, allowing for a proactive approach to reproductive health.

As we navigate the complexities of hormone health, it's clear that ovulation is not just a singular event but a cornerstone of the reproductive years. It's a dance of hormones, a convergence of timing, and a critical player in the journey from puberty to fertility. With this understanding, women can make informed decisions about their bodies, health, and futures.

Contraception and Hormonal Control

As we navigate the journey from puberty to fertility, it is equally important to discuss the choices available to women who wish to regulate their reproductive capabilities. Contraception and hormonal control are central to this discourse, offering women autonomy over their bodies and the freedom to decide if and when to have children.

Contraception comes in various forms, and hormonal methods are among the most popular and effective. These methods influence the natural hormonal rhythms that regulate ovulation and the menstrual cycle. Birth control pills, for instance, typically contain synthetic forms of estrogen and progesterone. By taking these hormones, a woman can prevent the release of an egg from her ovaries, thicken cervical mucus to block sperm, and thin the lining of the uterus to reduce the likelihood of implantation.

Another hormonal method includes the contraceptive patch, which releases hormones through the skin, and the vaginal ring, which releases hormones locally within the vagina. Both methods work similarly to the pill but offer convenience for those who prefer not to take a daily tablet.

Injectable contraceptives, such as the Depo-Provera shot, provide a longer-term solution, requiring administration every three months. The shot contains progestin, which suppresses ovulation and thickens cervical mucus.

For women seeking even longer-lasting contraception, hormonal implants and intrauterine devices (IUDs) can protect against pregnancy for several years. The implant, a tiny rod inserted under the skin of the arm, releases a steady dose of progestin. Hormonal IUDs, placed inside the uterus, release hormones locally to prevent fertilization.

While hormonal contraceptives are highly effective, they are not without potential side effects. Some women may experience changes in their menstrual cycle, mood swings, weight fluctuations, or other symptoms. It's essential to have an open dialogue with a healthcare provider to choose the most suitable method and to understand the possible effects on one's body and lifestyle.

Moreover, hormonal contraception can play a therapeutic role beyond birth control. For women with specific reproductive health issues, such as heavy menstrual bleeding, painful periods, or endometriosis, hormonal methods can offer significant relief. They regulate the menstrual cycle and can reduce the severity of symptoms, improving quality of life.

It is also important to acknowledge that while hormonal contraception can be empowering, it is not a one-size-fits-all solution. Each woman's body and hormonal balance are unique, and what works for one may not work for another. Personal preferences, health history, and future fertility plans are all critical factors in determining the best method of contraception.

In the next phase of our exploration into hormone health for women, we will delve into a condition that intimately ties into hormonal balance and reproductive health: Polycystic Ovary Syndrome (PCOS). This syndrome can affect a woman's hormonal levels, menstrual cycle, and overall health, and understanding its implications is vital for those who experience it.

Polycystic Ovary Syndrome: Insights and Management

In the journey of understanding hormone health for women, we've explored the nuances of contraception and hormonal control. Now we delve into a condition that intimately intertwines with these themes: Polycystic Ovary Syndrome, commonly known as PCOS. This syndrome is a complex endocrine disorder that affects an estimated one in ten women of reproductive age, making it a prevalent but often misunderstood condition.

PCOS is characterized by a combination of symptoms that can include irregular menstrual cycles, excess androgen levels (male hormones typically present in women in small amounts), and polycystic ovaries, which are enlarged and contain numerous small cysts. While the exact cause of PCOS remains unknown, it is believed to involve a combination of genetic and environmental factors, including insulin resistance and inflammation.

Women with PCOS often experience a range of symptoms that can vary in severity from mild to severe. These can include weight gain, acne, hirsutism (excessive hair growth on the face and body), thinning hair on the scalp, and difficulties with fertility. The emotional toll of managing these symptoms can be significant, leading to frustration and isolation.

Diagnosis of PCOS typically involves a review of medical history, physical examination, blood tests to measure hormone levels, and possibly an ultrasound to assess the ovaries. Because PCOS can mimic other health issues, it's crucial to rule out other potential causes of the symptoms.

Once diagnosed, management of PCOS is tailored to the individual's symptoms and concerns, such as managing irregular periods, acne, excess hair growth, and weight. Lifestyle changes, including diet and exercise, are pivotal in managing PCOS. A balanced diet rich in whole foods and low in processed carbohydrates can help manage insulin levels and support weight loss. Regular physical activity can also improve the body's sensitivity to insulin and aid in weight management.

For those struggling with fertility, medications that stimulate ovulation can be an option. Metformin, a medication commonly used to treat type 2 diabetes, has also been shown to improve insulin resistance in women with PCOS and can assist with ovulation.

Beyond physical symptoms, it's essential to address the psychological impact of PCOS. Support groups, counseling, and open dialogue with healthcare providers can provide invaluable emotional support. Women with PCOS may also face an increased risk for other health conditions, including type 2 diabetes, high blood pressure, and heart disease, making regular monitoring and preventive care essential.

In managing PCOS, the goal is not just to treat the symptoms but to empower women with the knowledge and resources they need to lead healthy, fulfilling lives. It's a journey that requires patience, understanding, and a compassionate approach to care. With the proper support and management strategies, women with PCOS can navigate the complexities of the condition and embrace their reproductive years with confidence and optimism.

Chapter Summary

- Puberty marks the beginning of a female's reproductive years, starting with hormonal changes and the onset of menstruation, typically between ages 8 and 13.
- The hypothalamus releases GnRH, which prompts the pituitary gland to produce FSH and LH, leading to egg maturation and hormone production in the ovaries.
- Estrogen is responsible for developing secondary sexual characteristics and preparing the uterus lining for potential pregnancy.
- The first menstrual cycles may be irregular and not involve ovulation, which is expected as the body adjusts its hormonal balance. Young women may experience mood swings, cramps, and other symptoms as they adjust to the hormonal changes during puberty. Open conversations and education about puberty can empower young women and promote a positive body image.
- The menstrual cycle, typically around 28 days, involves hormonal fluctuations that prepare the uterus for pregnancy and cause menstruation if no pregnancy occurs.
- Ovulation is the release of a mature egg, presenting a narrow window for fertilization; understanding this process is key for both conception and contraception.
- Hormonal contraceptives, like birth control pills, patches, rings, injections, implants, and IUDs, regulate ovulation and menstrual cycles, offering birth control and relief for specific reproductive health issues. Side effects of hormonal contraceptives can include menstrual changes and mood

swings, and personal health history should guide contraceptive choices.
- Polycystic Ovary Syndrome (PCOS) affects one in ten women. It involves symptoms like irregular periods, excess androgens, and polycystic ovaries, with management tailored to individual needs.
- Lifestyle changes, medications for ovulation, and insulin resistance management are essential for PCOS treatment, along with support for the emotional impact of the condition.

3

PREGNANCY AND HORMONES: THE MIRACLE OF LIFE

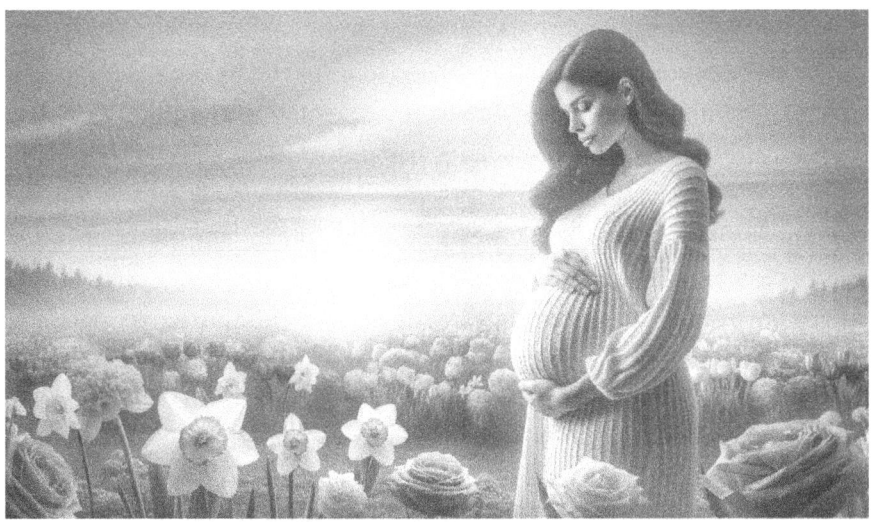

As we embark on this journey through the landscape of pregnancy, we'll begin to understand the profound hormonal shifts that occur within a woman's body. These changes are not just the backdrop to pregnancy; they are the very essence of it, orchestrating the development of new life with precision and care.

From the moment of conception, a woman's body becomes a finely tuned vessel for nurturing growth. The hormone human chorionic gonadotropin (hCG) is one of the first to enter the stage, signaling to the body that it's time to begin the incredible process of creating a new life. This hormone, produced by the cells that will eventually form the placenta, is responsible for maintaining the corpus luteum, which secretes progesterone to keep the uterine lining thick and hospitable for the embryo.

As the weeks progress, estrogen and progesterone levels rise dramatically. Progesterone, often referred to as the "pregnancy hormone," plays a critical role in relaxing the uterus muscles to prevent early contractions and stimulating the growth of blood vessels in the uterine lining to support the developing fetus. Estrogen, meanwhile, aids in the development of the placenta and stimulates the growth of the uterus itself.

Another key player is relaxin, a hormone that lives up to its name by relaxing the ligaments in the pelvis and softening and widening the cervix in preparation for childbirth. While its effects are most notable towards the end of pregnancy, relaxin begins to circulate early on. It is vital for the adjustments a woman's body must make to accommodate a growing baby.

The symphony of hormones during pregnancy also includes oxytocin, which is often associated with labor as it induces contractions of the uterus. However, its role extends beyond childbirth; oxytocin also fosters the bond between mother and child and plays a part in the milk ejection reflex during breastfeeding.

Pregnancy is a time of heightened sensitivity and responsiveness to hormonal signals; these are just a few key players. Each hormone has a specific and crucial role, ensuring that the environment within the womb is ideally suited to the needs of the developing fetus. The balance and levels of these hormones are meticulously regulated, as even the slightest deviation can affect the health and development of both mother and child.

As we delve deeper into the role of hormones in fetal development, we'll explore how these chemical messengers not only support the growth and nourishment of the fetus but also prepare the mother's body for the act of giving birth and the subsequent journey of motherhood. The intricate dance of hormones during pregnancy is nothing short of miraculous, reflecting the body's innate wisdom in fostering new life.

The Role of Hormones in Fetal Development

As we delve into the intricate dance of hormones during the gestational journey, it's essential to understand their pivotal role in developing a new life. From the moment of conception, a woman's body becomes a finely tuned orchestra of hormones, each with a specific part to play in the symphony of fetal development.

The first and perhaps most renowned of these hormonal players is human chorionic gonadotropin (hCG). This hormone is the chemical beacon that signals a positive result on a pregnancy test. But its role extends far beyond that initial announcement. hCG ensures the corpus luteum—remnants of the follicle that released the egg—continues to secrete progesterone and estrogen, vital in maintaining the uterine lining and setting the stage for the embryo's implantation and nourishment.

Progesterone, often called the "pregnancy hormone," takes on the crucial task of keeping the uterine lining healthy and thick, creating a supportive environment for the embryo. It also relaxes the uterus muscles, preventing contractions that could disrupt the pregnancy. As the placenta grows, it takes over progesterone production, steadily increasing its levels to adapt to the fetus's needs.

Estrogen, another critical hormone, rises alongside progesterone. It stimulates blood flow to the womb and fosters the growth of the placenta, ensuring the fetus receives the oxygen and nutrients essential for development. Estrogen also plays a role in developing the breast's milk ducts, preparing the body for the nurturing phase post-birth.

The placenta, an organ unique to pregnancy, acts not only as a nourishment conduit but also as an endocrine powerhouse, producing various hormones that support fetal growth and prepare the mother's body for childbirth. One such hormone is human placental lactogen (hPL), which helps to regulate the mother's metabolism and ensures that the growing fetus has an adequate supply of nutrients.

As the fetus develops, its tiny endocrine system begins to shape. The fetal adrenal glands produce dehydroepiandrosterone (DHEA), which the placenta converts into estrogen, further supporting the pregnancy. The fetal thyroid gland also starts to function, producing thyroid hormones critical for brain development and growth regulation.

The interplay of these hormones is a delicate balance, a testament to the body's innate wisdom. Each hormonal shift is like a brushstroke in the masterpiece of human development, painting the picture of a new life in the womb's protective canvas.

Understanding the hormonal milieu of pregnancy not only highlights the marvel of life's beginnings but also underscores the importance of supporting hormonal health throughout this transformative period. As we move forward, we'll explore how to navigate and manage these hormonal fluctuations to foster a healthy pregnancy for both mother and child.

Managing Hormonal Fluctuations in Pregnancy

As it embarks on the pregnancy journey, the body becomes a symphony of hormones, each playing a vital role in supporting your health and the development of a child. Understanding and managing these hormonal fluctuations can help to create a smoother pregnancy experience.

Estrogen and progesterone are the stars of this hormonal ballet, rising steadily to create a nurturing environment for the baby. These hormones, while essential, can also stir up a whirlwind of changes in the body, affecting everything from your mood to your metabolism.

One of the most common experiences during pregnancy is the emotional rollercoaster that can come with these hormonal shifts. One might find themselves feeling joyous one moment and tearful the next, often without a clear trigger. This is perfectly normal, and giving yourself grace during these times is essential. Communicating openly with your partner, family, and friends about what you're going through can help them provide the support you need.

Physical symptoms like nausea, often referred to as morning sickness, can also be a byproduct of hormonal changes. While it's typically more pronounced during the first trimester, it can persist or come and go throughout pregnancy. Eating small, frequent meals and staying hydrated can help manage these symptoms. Ginger tea and acupressure wristbands are also natural remedies that some women find helpful.

As the body adapts to its new hormonal milieu, one might notice changes in their skin and hair. The 'pregnancy glow' is not a myth; it results from increased blood flow and oil production. However, this can also lead to acne or other skin changes. Using gentle, non-comedogenic skincare products can help maintain skin health. Similarly, while some women enjoy thicker, more lustrous hair during pregnancy, others might experience hair thinning or changes in texture. A balanced diet and proper hair care can mitigate these effects.

Sleep patterns can be disrupted by hormonal fluctuations as well. Progesterone, in particular, can make you feel more fatigued. Creating a calming bedtime routine and ensuring a comfortable sleeping environment can aid in better sleep. Don't hesitate to use pillows to support your changing body.

It's also essential to monitor and manage any hormonal-related health concerns, such as gestational diabetes or preeclampsia, with the guidance of a healthcare provider. Regular prenatal visits are crucial for tracking hormone levels and health during pregnancy.

Remember, while these hormonal changes are temporary, their impact on the body and mind can be significant. It's okay to seek help and advice, whether from healthcare professionals, support groups, or your personal network. Your well-being is as important as the healthy development of the baby, and taking care of yourself is the first step in taking care of your little one.

Keep in mind that each woman's experience with pregnancy is unique. What works for one may not work for another, so listening to your body and finding what brings you comfort and health is important.

With understanding and care, you can manage these hormonal fluctuations and embrace the miracle of life unfolding within you.

Postpartum Hormonal Adjustments

As the journey of pregnancy culminates in the marvel of childbirth, a woman's body embarks on a new chapter of transformation. The postpartum period, often called the fourth trimester, is a time of immense hormonal shifts as the body transitions from pregnancy to its non-pregnant state. Understanding these hormonal adjustments can be helpful for new mothers navigating the postpartum period.

Immediately after delivery, the levels of pregnancy-related hormones such as estrogen and progesterone plummet. This sudden drop is a biological signal that you are no longer pregnant and triggers various physical and emotional responses. For instance, it's not uncommon for new mothers to experience a rollercoaster of emotions, often referred to as the "baby blues," which can include mood swings, weepiness, and feelings of overwhelm. These are typically short-lived, lasting a few days to a few weeks after delivery.

Another significant hormonal change involves the hormone prolactin, which rises during pregnancy and remains high if you are breastfeeding. Prolactin is responsible for milk production and affects mood and libido. Oxytocin, known as the love hormone, is also pivotal during this time. It facilitates bonding with your newborn and stimulates uterine contractions that help the uterus return to its pre-pregnancy size.

The thyroid gland can also be affected postpartum. Some women may experience postpartum thyroiditis, which can present with symptoms of both hyperthyroidism and hypothyroidism. This condition usually resolves independently, but it's important to be aware of the symptoms and seek medical advice if you suspect thyroid dysfunction.

It's essential to acknowledge that every woman's experience with postpartum hormonal adjustments is unique. While some may navigate this period relatively easily, others may find it more challenging. If you find yourself struggling with persistent mood changes, excessive fatigue, or other symptoms that concern you, it's important to reach out to your healthcare provider. Postpartum depression is a serious condition that affects many women and requires medical attention.

Remember that the body also adapts to a new normal during this time. Patience and self-care are key. Rest when you can, nourish your body with healthy foods, and don't hesitate to ask for support from loved ones or professionals. Your hormone levels will gradually stabilize, but giving yourself grace during this adjustment period is essential.

In the next part of our journey through hormone health, we'll explore the hormonal effects of breastfeeding, which not only nurtures a newborn but also continues to influence the postpartum hormonal landscape.

Breastfeeding and Hormonal Effects

As the journey of motherhood continues beyond the arrival of a child, the act of breastfeeding ushers in a new chapter of hormonal interplay that is as complex as it is beautiful. This natural process is not only about nourishment; it's a symphony of hormonal signals that fosters bonding, supports a baby's development, and subtly readies the body for potential future pregnancies.

A cascade of hormonal activity is triggered when a baby latches onto the breast. The primary hormones involved in breastfeeding are prolactin and oxytocin. Prolactin, often referred to as the 'milk-making hormone,' rises during pregnancy and reaches its peak after delivery. It is responsible for producing breast milk and ensures a steady supply for as long as you choose to nurse: each time a baby feeds, prolactin levels in the body rise, reinforcing the milk production cycle.

Oxytocin, fondly known as the 'love hormone,' plays a pivotal role in the let-down reflex – a critical response where the milk is released from the alveoli, tiny sacs within the breast, into the milk ducts where a nursing infant can access it. This hormone facilitates bonding between mother and child and has calming effects on both. The physical closeness and skin-to-skin contact during breastfeeding further enhance the release of oxytocin, strengthening the emotional connection and providing a sense of peace and contentment.

Breastfeeding also has a significant impact on the menstrual cycle and fertility. The high levels of prolactin suppress the release of the hormones required for ovulation. This natural suppression can lead to lactational amenorrhea, a period during which menstruation is absent, providing a form of natural, though not entirely reliable, contraception known as the Lactational Amenorrhea Method (LAM). It's important to note that the return of fertility can vary significantly among women, and ovulation can occur even before the first postpartum period, so additional forms of contraception should be considered if avoiding pregnancy is the goal.

The hormonal effects of breastfeeding extend beyond the immediate postpartum period. Nursing can influence the return to pre-pregnancy weight, as lactation burns additional calories. It may also confer long-term health benefits, such as a reduced risk of certain breast and ovarian cancers. These protective effects are thought to be linked to the hormonal changes induced by breastfeeding, including the extended periods of low estrogen levels associated with lactational amenorrhea.

It's essential to acknowledge that while breastfeeding is a natural process, it's not always easy. Hormonal fluctuations, alongside physical and emotional challenges, can sometimes make breastfeeding a complex journey. Some women may experience difficulties with milk supply, latch, or other issues that can lead to feelings of frustration or inadequacy. It's crucial to seek support from healthcare providers, lactation consultants, and breastfeeding support groups, as they can offer guidance and reassurance during this time.

In the grand landscape of hormone health for women, breastfeeding is a remarkable period where the body's innate wisdom shines through. It's a time of profound transformation, not only for the baby, who thrives on the nourishment and comfort provided but also for the mother, whose body continues to amaze with its ability to adapt and nurture life in its most tender stages.

Chapter Summary

- Hormonal changes during pregnancy are normal, and orchestrate the development of new life with precision and care.
- Understanding and managing hormonal fluctuations during pregnancy can help create a smoother experience, addressing emotional changes, physical symptoms, and sleep disruptions.
- Human chorionic gonadotropin (hCG) is one of the first hormones in pregnancy, maintaining the corpus luteum and supporting the uterine lining.
- Progesterone, the "pregnancy hormone," relaxes the uterus muscles and stimulates blood vessel growth, while estrogen aids placenta development and uterus growth.
- Relaxin softens the pelvis ligaments and cervix, and oxytocin induces labor contractions and fosters mother-child bonding.
- The placenta acts as an endocrine organ, producing hormones like human placental lactogen (hPL) to regulate the mother's metabolism and support fetal growth.
- Fetal adrenal glands and thyroid contribute to hormone production, influencing estrogen levels and critical development.
- Postpartum hormonal adjustments involve a drop in pregnancy hormones, changes in mood, and the continuation of prolactin and oxytocin for breastfeeding and bonding.

4

PERIMENOPAUSE AND MENOPAUSE: TRANSITIONING PHASES

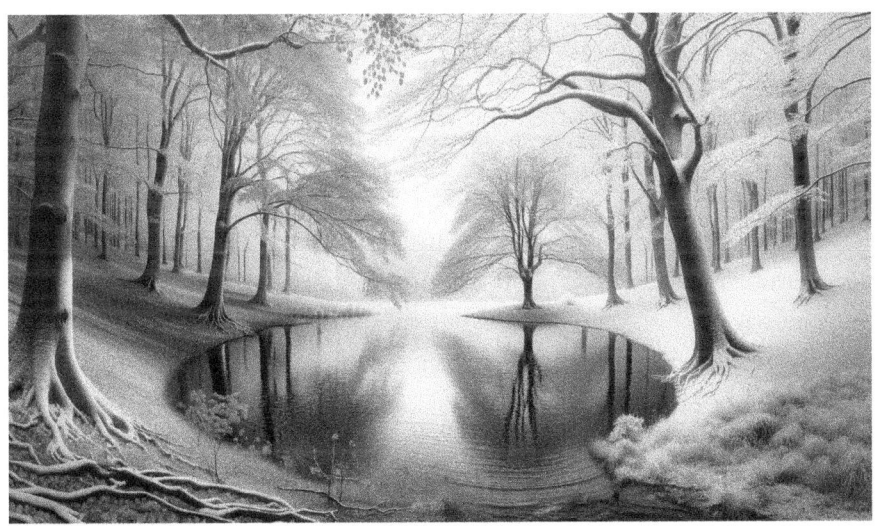

As the sun dips below the horizon, signaling the end of day and the beginning of twilight, so too does a woman's reproductive system signal its own transition. This natural shift is known as perimenopause. This term might be familiar, but its contours and nuances often remain shrouded in mystery. It's the prelude to a significant change when the body begins to compose a new narrative of hormone health.

Perimenopause typically commences in a woman's 40s, but for some, it can start as early as their 30s or as late as their 50s. It's a highly individual experience with a timeline spanning several years. During this phase, the ovaries gradually wind down their reproductive functions, producing less estrogen and progesterone—the hormones that have regulated menstruation and ovulation throughout a woman's life.

The ebb and flow of these hormones can be likened to the unpredictable patterns of the sea. Some days, the waters are calm, and on others, they are tumultuous. Women may notice that their menstrual cycles become irregular; periods may be heavier or lighter, longer or shorter, or they may skip a cycle entirely. This unpredictability is a hallmark of perimenopause and can be disconcerting. Still, it's important to remember that it's a normal part of the transition.

Beyond menstrual irregularity, other whispers of change may be felt. Some women experience hot flashes, those sudden waves of heat that wash over the body, often accompanied by a flushed face and sweating. Others might wake in the middle of the night, drenched in sweat—a nocturnal counterpart to hot flashes known as night sweats. These temperature irregularities are the body's response to the shifting sands of hormone levels.

Sleep disturbances during perimenopause are not limited to night sweats. The hormonal fluctuations can also lead to insomnia or restless sleep, making it difficult to get the restorative rest crucial to well-being. Mood swings may weave their way into daily life, with emotions swinging like a pendulum from joy to irritability or from energy to fatigue without a moment's notice.

It's not uncommon for women to notice changes in their sexual health during this time. Vaginal dryness and a decrease in libido can occur, which may affect intimacy and sexual relationships. These symptoms are rooted in the body's hormonal adjustments and are a normal part of the transition.

For some, perimenopause can also bring about a sense of loss or a challenge to their identity. The end of reproductive capability can evoke various emotions, from relief to sadness. It's important to acknowledge these feelings and understand that they are a natural response to change.

As we explore the waters of perimenopause, it's essential to remember that this is a time of transformation, not a disease to be cured. It's an opportunity to tune in to the body's signals and to care for oneself with compassion and understanding. Regular exercise, a balanced diet, stress management techniques, and open communication with healthcare providers and loved ones can all be part of a supportive strategy during this transition.

Perimenopause is the prelude to change, a time of preparation for the next stage of life's symphony. As we close this section, we carry with us the knowledge that while the body is shifting, it is also opening the door to a new phase of life—one that holds its unique beauty and challenges.

Understanding Menopause: Symptoms and Signs

As we navigate through the natural journey of hormonal shifts, understanding the signs and symptoms of menopause is like learning a new language spoken by our own bodies. This language, though at times seemingly foreign, is rich with information that can guide us toward self-care and informed choices.

Menopause, the cessation of menstruation for twelve consecutive months, is a natural biological process, not a medical condition. It marks the end of a woman's reproductive years, typically in the late 40s to early 50s. However, the experience of menopause is as unique as the individual, with symptoms varying widely in both type and intensity.

One of the most talked-about signs of menopause is the hot flash—a sudden warmth that spreads over the body, often most intense over the face, neck, and chest. These can be accompanied by sweating and sometimes followed by a chill. While the exact cause of hot flashes is not fully understood, they are thought to be related to the changes in hormone levels affecting the body's temperature regulation.

Night sweats, the nocturnal counterpart to hot flashes, can disrupt sleep and lead to insomnia. The importance of sleep for overall health cannot be overstated, so managing these symptoms is crucial. Many women find relief through lifestyle adjustments such as maintaining a cool sleeping environment and avoiding triggers like spicy foods or stress.

Irregular periods are another hallmark of the transition into menopause. You may notice changes in your menstrual cycle's frequency, duration, and flow. This unpredictability can be frustrating and sometimes alarming, but it's a normal part of the transition.

Vaginal dryness and discomfort during intercourse can occur as estrogen levels decline. These changes can affect sexual health and intimacy, but there are effective treatments and personal lubricants that can offer relief.

Emotional changes are also part of the menopause experience for many women. Mood swings, irritability, and feelings of sadness can be attributed to hormonal fluctuations, but they can also stem from the stress of dealing with other symptoms or life changes that often occur during this time.

Cognitive changes, such as difficulty concentrating and memory lapses, colloquially referred to as "menopause brain," can be concerning. It's important to note that these symptoms are usually temporary and can be mitigated through various strategies, including mental exercises and stress reduction techniques.

Physical changes are also evident during menopause. Many women experience a slowing metabolism and changes in weight distribution, often leading to weight gain around the abdomen. Maintaining a healthy diet and regular exercise routine can help manage these changes.

It's also a time to pay closer attention to bone health, as declining estrogen levels can decrease bone density, increasing the risk of osteoporosis. Calcium, vitamin D intake, and weight-bearing exercises are important preventive measures.

While these symptoms can be challenging, they are a natural part of the aging process. It's essential to approach this phase with self-compassion and to seek support from healthcare providers, friends, and family. Remember, menopause is not an end but a transition to a new phase of life that can be embraced with grace and resilience.

Hormone Replacement Therapy: Pros and Cons

As we navigate the transformative journey of perimenopause and menopause, many women consider various strategies to manage the symptoms that accompany these natural phases of life. One of the most discussed options is Hormone Replacement Therapy (HRT), which aims to replenish the body with estrogen and, in some cases, progesterone, which are no longer being produced at the levels they once were. The decision to use HRT is highly personal. It should be made with a thorough understanding of its potential benefits and risks.

On the positive side, HRT has been shown to be highly effective in alleviating some of the most common and uncomfortable symptoms of menopause, such as hot flashes, night sweats, vaginal dryness, and mood swings. By restoring hormone levels, HRT can also help prevent bone loss and reduce the risk of osteoporosis, a significant concern for many women as they age. Additionally, some studies suggest that HRT may offer some protection against heart disease when started early in the postmenopausal period.

However, the use of HRT is not without its controversies and potential drawbacks. The most significant concerns arise from studies that have linked the long-term use of certain types of HRT to an increased risk of breast cancer, blood clots, stroke, and heart disease. It's important to note that the risk varies depending on individual health factors, the type of hormones used, and the duration of therapy. For some women, particularly those with a family history of these conditions, the risks of HRT may outweigh the benefits.

Another consideration is the timing and duration of HRT. Research indicates that the window of opportunity for the potential benefits of HRT, particularly concerning heart health, may be limited to the early years of menopause. Furthermore, the current medical consensus generally recommends using the lowest effective dose for the shortest period necessary to manage symptoms.

It's also essential to recognize that HRT is not a one-size-fits-all solution. Women's bodies and responses to hormonal changes are as unique as their life stories. Therefore, the decision to use HRT should be made in close consultation with a healthcare provider, taking into account personal health history, family history, lifestyle, and the severity of menopausal symptoms.

For those who are candidates for HRT, there are various forms available, including pills, patches, gels, and creams. Each method has pros and cons, and what works for one woman may not be the best choice for another. It's a process of personalization and, sometimes, trial and error to find the most suitable and effective form of therapy.

In conclusion, while HRT can be a powerful tool in the management of menopausal symptoms and the prevention of specific long-term health issues, it is not a decision to be taken lightly. It requires a thoughtful conversation with a healthcare provider, a clear understanding of personal health risks, and a commitment to ongoing monitoring and adjustment. For those who decide that HRT is not the right choice or for those seeking complementary strategies, there are natural approaches to managing menopausal symptoms that can also offer relief and support during this phase of life.

Natural Approaches to Menopausal Symptoms

As we navigate the journey of perimenopause and menopause, it's essential to acknowledge that each woman's experience is as unique as she is. While hormone replacement therapy (HRT) has been discussed as one option for managing symptoms, many women seek natural approaches to find relief and support their bodies during this transition. Let's explore some natural strategies that can help ease the menopausal journey.

Lifestyle modifications are often the first line of defense. Regular physical activity is not only good for your heart and bones. Still, it can also help reduce hot flashes and improve mood. Aim for at least 150 minutes of moderate aerobic activity per week, complemented by strength training exercises. Yoga and tai chi, in particular, can be beneficial for stress reduction and improving balance, which can be affected during menopause.

The diet also plays a crucial role in managing menopausal symptoms. Foods rich in phytoestrogens, such as soybeans, flaxseeds, and certain whole grains, may offer a natural way to balance hormones. These plant-based compounds can mimic the effects of estrogen in the body, potentially easing hot flashes and other symptoms. However, it's essential to consult with a healthcare provider before making significant dietary changes, especially if you have any underlying health conditions.

Hydration is another crucial element. As simple as it sounds, drinking enough water can help with bloating and the dryness that often accompanies menopause. Aim for eight glasses daily, and consider adding hydrating foods like cucumbers and watermelon to your diet.

Sleep can become elusive during menopause, with night sweats and insomnia being common complaints. Creating a sleep-conducive environment, maintaining a regular bedtime routine, and possibly incorporating relaxation techniques like meditation or deep breathing exercises can be helpful. Some women find relief in natural supplements like melatonin, but it's important to discuss this with a healthcare provider before starting any new supplement regimen.

Herbal remedies have been used for centuries to alleviate menopausal symptoms. Herbs such as black cohosh, red clover, and dong quai are popular. Still, scientific evidence on their effectiveness varies, and they can interact with medications. Always consult with a healthcare professional before trying herbal treatments.

Stress management is also vital. Chronic stress can exacerbate menopausal symptoms, so finding effective ways to relax and decompress is essential. Mindfulness, therapy, or simply carving out time for hobbies and activities you enjoy can make a significant difference in your overall well-being.

Lastly, social support cannot be underestimated. Connecting with other women who are going through similar experiences can provide comfort and valuable insights. Whether through support groups, online forums, or just chatting with friends, sharing your journey can be incredibly therapeutic.

Remember, these natural approaches aim not just to treat symptoms but to enhance overall health and quality of life during menopause. It's about finding what works for you and making adjustments as needed, always in consultation with healthcare professionals who understand your health history and needs.

As we continue to explore the facets of hormone health for women, it's clear that the interplay between hormones and various aspects of health is complex. Next, we'll delve into the relationship between hormones and bone health, a critical consideration for aging women who want to maintain strength and vitality through menopause.

Bone Health and Hormones in Aging Women

As we gracefully navigate the waves of perimenopause and menopause, it's crucial to shine a light on an aspect of our health that often goes unnoticed until it demands our attention: our bones. Bone health is a silent but significant concern for aging women, and it's intimately tied to the hormonal changes that occur during this time.

Our bones are living tissues that constantly break down and rebuild. This process is regulated by hormones, including estrogen, which plays a pivotal role in maintaining bone density. During the fertile years, estrogen helps keep bone breakdown and rebuilding in balance. However, as we approach perimenopause and transition into menopause, estrogen levels begin to fluctuate and ultimately decline. This decline can accelerate bone loss, increasing the risk of osteoporosis—a condition where bones become weak and brittle.

Understanding the connection between hormones and bone health is the first step in taking proactive measures to protect and strengthen our skeletal framework. It's not just about preventing fractures; it's about maintaining a quality of life that allows us to continue the activities we love and live without the fear of injury.

So, what can we do to support our bone health during these years of change? Nutrition is a cornerstone. A diet rich in calcium and vitamin D is essential for bone strength. Calcium is a building block for bones, while vitamin D helps our bodies absorb calcium effectively. However, it's not just about the intake of these nutrients; it's also about how well our bodies can utilize them. Factors such as vitamin K2 and magnesium also play roles in bone health, helping to ensure calcium is deposited in our bones rather than in other tissues that can cause harm.

Physical activity, particularly weight-bearing and resistance exercises, is another powerful tool in our bone health arsenal. These activities improve strength and balance, reduce the risk of falls, and stimulate bone formation. Even simple activities like walking, dancing, or lifting weights can make a significant difference.

For some women, hormone replacement therapy (HRT) may be a consideration to help mitigate bone loss. It's a decision that should be made in close consultation with a healthcare provider, weighing the benefits against potential risks. HRT isn't suitable for everyone, but it can be an effective part of a comprehensive bone health strategy for certain individuals.

Addressing lifestyle factors that can negatively impact bone health is important. Smoking and excessive alcohol consumption can both contribute to bone loss, so taking steps to quit smoking and moderate alcohol intake can be beneficial. Additionally, being mindful of medications that may affect bone density, such as long-term use of steroids, is essential.

Lastly, regular screenings can play a critical role in maintaining bone health. Bone density tests, such as DEXA scans, can help detect osteoporosis before a fracture occurs, allowing for early intervention. These screenings are crucial for women with risk factors for osteoporosis, such as a family history of the condition, a petite body frame, or certain medical conditions and treatments.

The transition through perimenopause and menopause calls for a renewed commitment to our overall well-being, with bone health being a vital component. By understanding the hormonal shifts that occur and their impact on our bones, we can take informed and practical steps to ensure that our skeletal health supports us as we move through these chapters of life with strength and vitality.

Chapter Summary

- Perimenopause marks the beginning of the transition in a woman's reproductive system, typically starting in the 40s but can vary widely.
- During perimenopause, ovaries produce less estrogen and progesterone, leading to irregular menstrual cycles and symptoms like hot flashes and night sweats.
- Women may experience sleep disturbances, mood swings, and changes in sexual health, including vaginal dryness and decreased libido. The transition can evoke various emotions, from relief to sadness, as women come to terms with the end of their reproductive years.
- Menopause is the cessation of menstruation for twelve consecutive months, usually occurring in the late 40s to early 50s, with widespread symptoms.
- Common menopause symptoms include hot flashes, night sweats, irregular periods, vaginal dryness, emotional changes, cognitive challenges, and physical changes like weight gain.
- Hormone Replacement Therapy can alleviate menopausal symptoms and prevent bone loss but carries risks such as increased chances of breast cancer and heart disease.
- Natural approaches to managing menopausal symptoms include lifestyle changes, diet, hydration, sleep management, herbal remedies, stress management, and social support.

- Bone health is crucial during perimenopause and menopause due to declining estrogen levels, with nutrition and physical activity vital to maintaining bone density.
- Hormone Replacement Therapy may be considered for bone health. Lifestyle factors like smoking and alcohol consumption should be managed, and regular bone density screenings are recommended.

5

THYROID HEALTH: THE METABOLIC REGULATOR

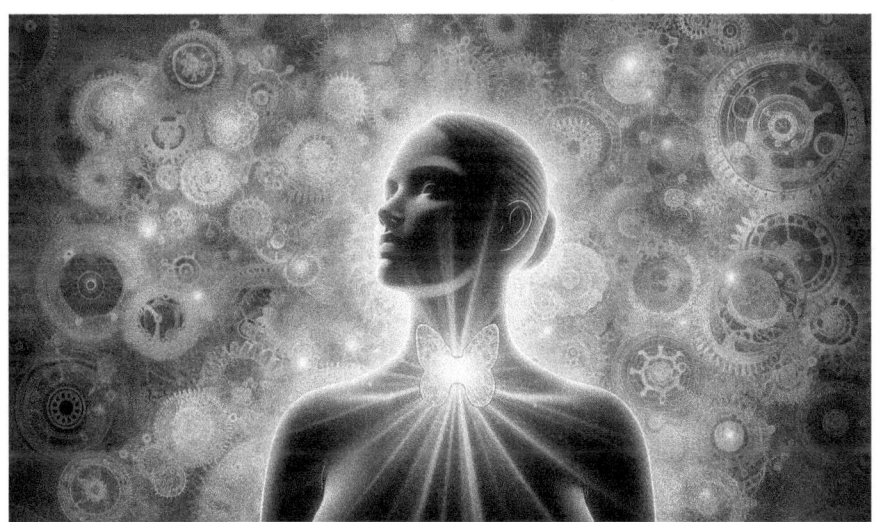

Nestled at the base of your neck, the thyroid gland may be small, but its impact on your body is mighty. This butterfly-shaped gland is the maestro of your metabolism, conducting the symphony of hormones that regulate how your body uses energy.

Understanding how your thyroid functions is like uncovering the secret to how your body's cells dance to the rhythm of life.

The thyroid produces two main hormones: thyroxine (T4) and triiodothyronine (T3). These hormones travel through your bloodstream and reach nearly every cell, influencing multiple functions such as your heart rate, body temperature, and how quickly you burn calories. It's a delicate balance, and when it's just right, you feel like you're on top of the world—energized, focused, and balanced.

But what happens when this balance is disrupted? Imagine a car with a sputtering engine or a clock that ticks too slowly. That's akin to what your body experiences when the thyroid isn't producing enough hormones—a condition known as hypothyroidism. It's like the conductor of your metabolic orchestra has suddenly slowed the tempo, and every musician (or cell) is struggling to keep up.

The thyroid's ability to produce these vital hormones hinges on a complex feedback loop involving the hypothalamus and the pituitary gland, two key players in your brain. The hypothalamus releases thyrotropin-releasing hormone (TRH), which prompts the pituitary gland to produce thyroid-stimulating hormone (TSH). TSH then signals to the thyroid how much T4 and T3 should be released into the bloodstream. It's a finely tuned system; when it works well, it's seamless and unnoticeable. But when it doesn't, the effects on your body and well-being can be profound.

For women, maintaining thyroid health is particularly crucial. The ebb and flow of female hormones can influence thyroid function, and various stages of a woman's life—such as puberty, pregnancy, and menopause—can change thyroid hormone levels. It's not uncommon for women to first notice symptoms of a thyroid imbalance during these times of hormonal fluctuation.

So, how do you know if your thyroid is not performing its role as it should? It starts with tuning into your body and recognizing the signs that may indicate your thyroid is underactive. In the next section, we'll delve into hypothyroidism, exploring what happens when your thyroid slows down, the symptoms to watch for, and how this condition can affect your overall health. It's a journey into understanding the subtler aspects of your body's internal workings, and with knowledge comes the power to seek harmony within.

Hypothyroidism: When the Thyroid Slows Down

In the intricate dance of hormones that governs our well-being, the thyroid gland plays a pivotal role, orchestrating many bodily functions with the precision of a seasoned conductor. When this gland's activity diminishes, a condition known as hypothyroidism emerges, casting a wide net over one's health and vitality.

Hypothyroidism is akin to a slow-burning flame, often starting so subtly that it's easily dismissed or mistaken for the wear and tear of daily life. Women, in particular, may notice a gradual onset of fatigue that no amount of sleep seems to alleviate. It's as if the body's internal battery is perpetually low, no matter how long it's been on charge.

But fatigue is just the tip of the iceberg. With hypothyroidism, the metabolism—the body's engine for burning calories—downshifts. Weight gain may occur, even when eating habits haven't changed. The skin, once supple, may become dry and cool to the touch, while hair that was once lustrous and full may turn brittle and thin. These physical changes are not merely cosmetic but external manifestations of an internal imbalance.

The thyroid's influence extends to the very rhythm of our hearts. A slower heartbeat can be a sign of an underactive thyroid, as can an increase in blood cholesterol levels, which is why hypothyroidism is often discovered during routine health screenings.

For women, the menstrual cycle is a delicate interplay of hormones, and the thyroid is a key player. An underactive thyroid can lead to heavier, more frequent, and more painful periods. It can also be a stealthy saboteur of fertility, often overlooked in the quest to conceive.

The mental and emotional realms are not immune to the thyroid's reach. Hypothyroidism can cloud the mind, making concentration difficult and memory elusive. It can also cast a shadow over one's mood, contributing to feelings of depression or a pervasive sense of malaise.

Diagnosing hypothyroidism involves a careful evaluation of symptoms and blood tests that measure thyroid hormone levels. The most common treatment is a daily dose of synthetic thyroid hormone, which replaces what the body can no longer produce in sufficient quantities. This medication, typically a lifelong commitment, is a beacon of hope for many, often restoring energy levels and normalizing bodily functions.

Living with hypothyroidism is a journey of balance and awareness. It requires tuning in to the body's signals and working closely with healthcare providers to fine-tune treatment. It's about understanding that this small gland, nestled in the neck, holds great power over the symphony of hormones that animate our lives.

As we navigate the complexities of hormone health, it's essential to remember that each person's experience with hypothyroidism is unique. Patience and self-compassion become vital companions on the path to wellness, reminding us that the journey is as much about nurturing the spirit as it is about treating the body.

Hyperthyroidism: The Overactive Thyroid

In the intricate dance of hormones that governs our well-being, the thyroid gland often takes center stage, especially for women. When it becomes overactive—a condition known as hyperthyroidism—it can lead to a symphony of symptoms that disrupt the rhythm of daily life.

Hyperthyroidism occurs when the thyroid gland produces too much of the hormones thyroxine (T4) and triiodothyronine (T3). Excessive amounts of these hormones accelerate bodily functions, leading to various signs and symptoms.

Imagine your body as a car. With hyperthyroidism, it's as if the thyroid is pushing the accelerator too hard. You might experience a rapid or irregular heartbeat, a sensation that your heart is pounding (palpitations), and even the feeling of being on edge or nervous. These are the telltale signs that your body is running on overdrive.

Weight loss is another familiar hallmark of hyperthyroidism, even when your appetite and food intake remain the same or increase. It can be puzzling and distressing to lose weight without trying, and it's often what prompts many women to seek medical advice. Alongside this, you may notice increased sweating, sensitivity to heat, and a more frequent need to quench your thirst.

For women, menstrual cycles can become lighter and less frequent. This disruption to the menstrual cycle is not only a concern for overall health but can also affect fertility. It reminds us how closely our reproductive health is linked to proper thyroid functioning.

Changes in mood and mental state can accompany the physical changes. You might feel unusually anxious, irritable, or having difficulty concentrating. Sleep can become elusive despite feeling tired, creating a frustrating cycle of fatigue and restlessness.

In some cases, you may notice a swelling at the base of your neck, which is a goiter. This is the thyroid gland becoming enlarged and can be a visual clue that something is amiss. While not all cases of hyperthyroidism result in noticeable goiters, their presence can exacerbate the feeling of tightness or discomfort in the throat, sometimes making swallowing a challenge.

The causes of hyperthyroidism are varied, with autoimmune disorders, nodules on the thyroid gland, and certain medications being among the common culprits. Understanding the underlying cause is crucial for effective treatment, which may include medication to reduce hormone production, radioactive iodine to shrink the gland, or even surgery in some cases.

Living with hyperthyroidism can be a delicate balancing act, requiring careful monitoring and often lifelong management. It's a journey that can sometimes feel overwhelming. Still, with the proper support and treatment, many women find a new equilibrium. The key is to listen to your body, advocate for your health, and work closely with healthcare professionals who understand the nuances of thyroid disorders.

As we navigate the complexities of thyroid health, it's important to remember that each woman's experience is unique. Whether you're dealing with the slowing down of hypothyroidism or the acceleration of hyperthyroidism, your story is your own. And while the path to managing thyroid conditions is not always straightforward, it's a path that leads to a deeper understanding of your body and its needs.

Autoimmune Thyroid Diseases: Hashimoto's and Graves'

The thyroid gland plays a pivotal role in orchestrating various metabolic processes in the intricate dance of the body's endocrine system. For many women, the harmony of this dance is disrupted by autoimmune thyroid diseases, which can lead to a cascade of health challenges. Two of the most common conditions are Hashimoto's thyroiditis and Graves' disease, each representing opposite ends of the thyroid function spectrum.

Hashimoto's thyroiditis is the most prevalent form of thyroid inflammation. It is often the underlying cause of hypothyroidism, a state in which the thyroid gland underproduces hormones. This condition is characterized by the immune system mistakenly attacking the thyroid, leading to damage and impaired hormone production. Women with Hashimoto's may experience a variety of symptoms, including fatigue, weight gain, cold intolerance, and muscle weakness, among others. The onset of Hashimoto's is typically gradual, and it may take years before the symptoms prompt a woman to seek medical attention.

Conversely, Graves' disease is an autoimmune disorder that leads to hyperthyroidism or an overactive thyroid. In Graves' disease, the immune system produces antibodies that bind to the thyroid gland, causing it to produce an excess of thyroid hormones. This overactivity can manifest in symptoms such as unexplained weight loss, rapid heartbeat, increased sweating, and anxiety. Unlike the slow progression of Hashimoto's, the symptoms of Graves' disease can emerge more abruptly. They can be more immediately disruptive to a woman's well-being.

Diagnosing these conditions typically involves a combination of blood tests to measure thyroid hormone levels and the presence of specific antibodies, along with a thorough clinical evaluation. Imaging studies like ultrasound or radioactive iodine uptake tests may also be employed to understand the thyroid's structure and function better.

Management of Hashimoto's and Graves' disease often requires a personalized approach, as the impact on each woman's body can vary greatly. For those with Hashimoto's, treatment usually involves hormone replacement therapy to restore normal thyroid hormone levels. In the case of Graves' disease, treatment options may include medications to inhibit hormone production, radioactive iodine therapy to reduce thyroid activity, or surgery in more severe cases.

Living with an autoimmune thyroid disease can be an emotional journey, as the symptoms can affect not only physical health but also emotional well-being and quality of life. It's important for women to have a supportive healthcare team that not only addresses the physiological aspects of the disease but also provides guidance on coping with the emotional and psychological impacts.

As we move forward, understanding the role of nutrition and lifestyle in supporting thyroid health becomes increasingly important. While medical treatments address physiological imbalances, integrating holistic practices can empower women to manage their condition and improve their overall well-being actively.

Nutrition and Lifestyle for Thyroid Health

In the intricate dance of hormones that governs a woman's health, the thyroid plays a pivotal role, orchestrating the tempo at which her body operates. The right nutrition and lifestyle choices can be influential conductors for this metabolic symphony, helping to maintain harmony and balance.

A well-rounded diet is essential when nourishing the thyroid, starting with the basics. This means embracing a variety of fruits and vegetables, which are rich in antioxidants and essential nutrients. These colorful foods are not just a feast for the eyes; they provide the vitamins and minerals your thyroid needs to function optimally.

Among these nutrients, iodine is a critical component for thyroid hormone production. While iodine deficiency is less common in many developed countries due to iodized salt, it's still important to include natural sources in your diet. Seaweed, fish, and dairy are excellent sources of iodine. Still, consuming them in moderation is vital to avoid an excess, which can be just as detrimental as a deficiency.

Selenium is another mineral that deserves a spotlight. It plays a crucial role in the conversion of thyroid hormones from their inactive to active forms. Foods like Brazil nuts, sunflower seeds, and whole grains are rich in selenium and can support thyroid health.

But it's not just about what you eat; it's also about how you eat. Stress can wreak havoc on your thyroid, and one way to combat this is through mindful eating. Taking the time to savor your food, eating slowly, and listening to your body's hunger cues can help manage stress levels and support overall well-being.

Physical activity is another cornerstone of a thyroid-friendly lifestyle. Regular exercise can help regulate thyroid function, boost mood, and improve energy levels. It doesn't have to be a high-intensity workout; even a daily walk or gentle yoga can make a significant difference.

Sleep, that often-neglected aspect of health, is also vital for thyroid function. Aim for 7-9 hours of quality sleep per night. Establishing a calming bedtime routine and ensuring your bedroom is a sanctuary can help you drift off to the restorative sleep your body—and thyroid—needs.

Lastly, avoiding certain substances that can interfere with thyroid function is important. Smoking, excessive alcohol consumption, and exposure to environmental toxins can all harm thyroid health. Being mindful of these factors and minimizing exposure can benefit your thyroid and overall health.

Remember, each woman's body is unique, and what works for one may not work for another. It's always wise to consult with a healthcare provider before significantly changing your diet or lifestyle, especially if you have a thyroid condition. They can provide personalized advice that takes into account your individual health needs.

By embracing these nutritional and lifestyle practices, you're not just supporting your thyroid but investing in your overall health and well-being. It's a journey of self-care that can lead to a more vibrant, balanced life.

Chapter Summary

- The thyroid gland, located at the base of the neck, is crucial for metabolism, producing hormones T4 and T3 that affect energy use in the body.
- Women's thyroid health is vital due to hormonal fluctuations during puberty, pregnancy, and menopause.
- Thyroid hormone imbalances can lead to hypothyroidism, where the body's functions slow down, or hyperthyroidism, where they speed up.
- Hypothyroidism symptoms include fatigue, weight gain, dry skin, slow heart rate, menstrual changes, and mental fog, and it's treated with synthetic hormones.
- Hyperthyroidism symptoms include rapid heartbeat, weight loss, heat sensitivity, menstrual changes, and anxiety, and it's treated with medication, radioactive iodine, or surgery.
- Autoimmune thyroid diseases like Hashimoto's thyroiditis (leading to hypothyroidism) and Graves' disease (leading to hyperthyroidism) affect the thyroid's function.
- Nutrition and lifestyle choices, such as a balanced diet rich in iodine and selenium, mindful eating, regular exercise, and adequate sleep, support thyroid health.
- Avoiding substances that interfere with thyroid function, like smoking and environmental toxins, is vital for maintaining thyroid and overall health.

6

STRESS AND HORMONES: THE ADRENAL CONNECTION

In the intricate dance of the body's response to stress, understanding the physiology is like learning the steps to a complex routine. It's a choreography that involves various organs and hormones, all working in tandem to help you navigate through the challenges that life throws your way.

The adrenal gland is at the heart of this dance, a small but mighty organ that sits atop your kidneys like a hat. When you encounter a stressful situation, your brain sends a signal to these glands, cueing them to release a cascade of hormones. These hormones are the body's equivalent of a backstage crew working behind the scenes to prepare you for action.

The initial response is almost instantaneous. Adrenaline, also known as epinephrine, floods your system, heightening your senses, quickening your pulse, and pumping more blood to your muscles. This is the 'fight or flight' response that our ancestors relied on for survival, and it's just as relevant today when we need to react swiftly to a potential threat or challenge.

But the stress response doesn't end there. After the initial surge of adrenaline, the adrenals release another hormone that plays a longer-term role in how your body manages stress. This hormone is cortisol, often referred to as the stress hormone, and it has a wide range of effects on your body.

Cortisol ensures that your body has enough energy to deal with prolonged stress. It does this by increasing glucose in the bloodstream, enhancing your brain's use of glucose, and increasing the availability of substances that repair tissues. Cortisol also curbs functions that would be nonessential or detrimental in a fight-or-flight situation. It alters immune system responses and suppresses the digestive system, the reproductive system, and growth processes.

This complex hormonal interplay is designed to be self-regulating. Once the perceived threat has passed, hormone levels should return to normal as part of the body's feedback mechanism. However, this system can become overtaxed in our modern world with its constant barrage of stressors. When stress becomes chronic, the adrenal glands may continue to produce cortisol at elevated levels. This can lead to a host of issues, as the body is constantly alert, never quite returning to its baseline.

Understanding the physiology of stress is crucial because it helps us recognize the importance of managing our stress response. It's not just about feeling less frazzled; it's about maintaining the delicate balance of our hormonal health. As we move forward, we'll delve deeper into cortisol, the stress hormone, and explore its profound impact on our bodies and well-being.

Cortisol: The Stress Hormone

In the intricate dance of hormones that affects every aspect of a woman's health, cortisol plays a lead role in stress. Often referred to as the "stress hormone," cortisol is produced by the adrenal glands, which are small but mighty organs perched atop your kidneys like vigilant sentinels. Understanding cortisol's function is crucial to comprehending how stress influences our bodies and, more specifically, its unique implications for women.

Cortisol is not a villain. In fact, it's essential for survival. It helps regulate various processes in the body, including metabolism and the immune response. It also has a pivotal role in helping the body respond to stress. When you encounter a stressful situation, your brain triggers the release of cortisol. This hormone then courses through your body, preparing you for the "fight or flight" response. It sharpens your senses, quickens your heartbeat, and releases energy stores to give you the necessary resources to handle the challenge at hand.

However, the story of cortisol is a tale of balance. While acute stress can lead to a temporary spike in cortisol, which is normal and often beneficial, the problems arise when stress becomes chronic. In today's fast-paced world, many women find themselves in a constant state of low-grade stress, whether it's due to work pressures, family responsibilities, health concerns, or social dynamics. This persistent stress can lead to a sustained high level of cortisol, which is where the trouble begins.

High cortisol levels over prolonged periods can adversely affect your health. It can disrupt sleep, lead to weight gain, increase blood pressure, and contribute to mood swings or feelings of anxiety. These effects can be particularly pronounced for women due to the interplay between cortisol and female sex hormones like estrogen and progesterone.

Moreover, the impact of sustained high cortisol can extend to menstrual cycles, potentially causing irregular periods or worsening symptoms of premenstrual syndrome (PMS). It can also play a role in the onset of menopause and the severity of its symptoms. During menopause, as the body's production of estrogen and progesterone decreases, the sensitivity to cortisol can increase, making stress management even more critical.

It's essential to recognize the signs that your body may be experiencing the adverse effects of too much cortisol. These can include fatigue, difficulty concentrating, and a general sense of being overwhelmed. By acknowledging these signals, you can take proactive steps to manage stress and, in turn, help regulate your cortisol levels.

Several strategies can help maintain healthy cortisol levels. Regular physical activity is one of the most effective, as it can boost mood and improve sleep, which can help modulate cortisol production. Mindfulness practices, such as meditation or deep breathing exercises, can be beneficial. Maintaining a balanced diet and ensuring adequate rest are critical components of a holistic approach to managing stress and supporting hormone health.

In essence, cortisol is a critical hormone that helps your body cope with stress but requires a delicate balance. Too much or too little can have significant implications for your overall well-being. Understanding cortisol's role and taking steps to manage stress can support your body's natural rhythms and promote hormone health, an essential part of a balanced and healthy life as a woman.

Adrenal Fatigue: Myth or Reality?

In the bustling rhythm of modern life, where stress often seems like a constant companion, the term "adrenal fatigue" has found a foothold in conversations about health and well-being, particularly among women. It's a phrase used to describe a collection of symptoms believed to be caused by a prolonged, overactive stress response that eventually wears down the adrenal glands, leading to exhaustion.

Recall that the small but mighty adrenal glands sit atop your kidneys like vigilant sentinels, orchestrating your body's reactions to stress through the release of hormones such as cortisol, which we've explored in depth. When life's demands become relentless, these glands are put through their paces, pumping out these hormones to help you navigate the challenges you face.

But what happens when the stress is unending when the alarm bells of your life never seem to quiet? This is where the concept of adrenal fatigue enters the conversation. It suggests that after long periods of chronic stress, the adrenal glands can no longer keep up with the body's demand for these regulatory hormones, leading to symptoms such as fatigue, sleep disturbances, weight gain, and a craving for salt or sugar.

However, it's important to approach this topic with a discerning eye. The medical community is divided on the existence of adrenal fatigue as a medical diagnosis. Conventional medicine does recognize conditions such as Addison's disease, where the adrenal glands produce insufficient hormones, and Cushing's syndrome, characterized by an overproduction. Yet, adrenal fatigue occupies a gray area, with many health professionals questioning its validity due to a lack of robust scientific evidence.

Despite this skepticism in some circles, there are countless women who identify with the symptoms attributed to adrenal fatigue. They seek answers and relief for their persistent tiredness and other related health concerns. It's essential to validate these experiences, acknowledging that while the term "adrenal fatigue" may not be widely accepted, the symptoms are very real to those suffering from them.

In navigating this complex issue, it's crucial to consider the physiological and psychological components of stress. The body's response to stress is intricate. It can affect various systems beyond the adrenals, including the digestive, immune, and nervous systems. Therefore, addressing stress-related symptoms often requires a holistic approach that looks at lifestyle, diet, sleep, exercise, and emotional well-being.

For those feeling the weight of these symptoms, the journey toward balance and health can be a personal one, filled with trial and error. It involves tuning into your body's signals, recognizing when to slow down, and finding strategies that help restore your sense of equilibrium. This journey is not about chasing a one-size-fits-all solution but discovering what works for your unique body and situation.

As we move forward, we'll delve into practical strategies that can help manage stress and support hormonal balance. These approaches aim to empower you with tools to enhance your resilience against the pressures of life, fostering a sense of well-being that is both sustainable and nurturing.

Strategies for Managing Stress and Hormonal Balance

Stress is often the leader in the intricate dance of hormone health, guiding the tempo and rhythm of our hormonal responses. Understanding this, we can choreograph a life-supporting balance and well-being. Let's explore strategies to help manage stress and maintain hormonal harmony.

First and foremost, nurturing a healthy diet is paramount. Foods rich in vitamins and minerals, such as leafy greens, nuts, seeds, and lean proteins, provide the nutrients necessary for adrenal support. Integrating complex carbohydrates like whole grains can help stabilize blood sugar levels, supporting adrenal health. Additionally, certain herbs such as ashwagandha and rhodiola have been traditionally used to help the body adapt to stress.

Regular physical activity is another cornerstone of stress management. Exercise not only helps to reduce the levels of stress hormones in the body but also boosts the production of endorphins, the body's natural mood elevators. Whether it's a brisk walk, a yoga session, or a dance class, finding an activity that brings joy can make exercise an enjoyable and effective stress reliever.

Mindfulness and relaxation techniques such as meditation, deep breathing exercises, and progressive muscle relaxation can also help manage stress. These practices help calm the mind and reduce the physiological effects of stress, promoting a sense of tranquility that supports hormonal balance.

Sleep is an often underestimated yet crucial component of hormonal health. Establishing a regular sleep routine and creating a restful environment can enhance the quality of sleep, which in turn can help regulate the production and release of stress hormones.

Lastly, fostering strong social connections and seeking support can provide emotional comfort and reduce stress. Whether talking with a friend, joining a support group, or seeking professional counseling, having a network to lean on is invaluable.

By incorporating these strategies into daily life, it's possible to create a foundation supporting hormonal health and overall well-being. Remember, the journey to balance is personal and unique to each individual. It's about finding what works for you and making small, sustainable changes that can lead to a healthier, more harmonious life.

Stress and Female Hormonal Disorders

Stress often steps on the toes of hormonal harmony, particularly for women. When stress enters the scene, the adrenal glands spring into action, secreting cortisol, the primary stress hormone. This response is part of the body's natural survival mechanism, the fight-or-flight response, which, in ancient times, was a crucial reaction to immediate threats.

However, the persistent stress of modern life doesn't come in the form of occasional predators but rather as a relentless stream of deadlines, social pressures, and multitasking demands. This constant state of alert can lead to an overproduction of cortisol, which, over time, can wreak havoc on the female body.

Cortisol's role is not inherently evil; it's essential for various bodily functions, including regulating metabolism, reducing inflammation, and assisting with memory formulation. But when stress is chronic, the sustained high levels of cortisol can lead to a cascade of female hormonal disorders.

One of the most significant impacts of prolonged stress is on the menstrual cycle. Cortisol can inhibit the production of gonadotropin-releasing hormone (GnRH), which is responsible for the release of the hormones that trigger ovulation and menstruation. This disruption can lead to irregular periods, anovulation, or even amenorrhea, the absence of menstruation.

Stress can also exacerbate premenstrual syndrome (PMS) and premenstrual dysphoric disorder (PMDD), conditions that affect a significant number of women. The delicate balance between estrogen and progesterone can be tipped by the scales of stress, leading to mood swings, bloating, and other symptoms that can range from mildly irritating to severely debilitating.

Furthermore, the relationship between stress and hormones extends to fertility. Chronic stress can impact fertility by affecting the hormones that are essential for conception. It can also influence libido, creating a challenging cycle for women who are trying to conceive, as stress about fertility can further impair hormonal balance and reproductive function.

The adrenal glands' overexertion doesn't stop with reproductive hormones. There's a complex interplay between cortisol and insulin, the hormone responsible for regulating blood sugar levels. High cortisol can lead to increased blood sugar, which, over time, can contribute to insulin resistance and the risk of developing type 2 diabetes.

Moreover, the adrenal glands' production of another hormone, DHEA (dehydroepiandrosterone), can be affected by stress. DHEA is involved in producing other hormones, including estrogen and testosterone. An imbalance in DHEA levels can lead to various symptoms, including fatigue, muscle loss, and decreased bone density, which are particularly concerning for women as they age.

The impact of stress on thyroid function is another critical aspect of the adrenal connection. The thyroid gland, which regulates metabolism, can be slowed down by high cortisol levels, leading to symptoms such as weight gain, fatigue, and depression.

Understanding the link between stress and female hormonal disorders is the first step toward restoring balance. It's not about eliminating stress—an unrealistic goal in our fast-paced world—but rather about managing the body's response to stress. By recognizing the signs of hormonal imbalance and taking proactive steps to mitigate stress, women can help safeguard their hormonal health and overall well-being.

In this journey toward hormonal equilibrium, it's essential to acknowledge that the body's signals are not just noise to be ignored but messages to be heeded. By tuning into these signals and responding with self-care, stress reduction techniques, and, when necessary, medical intervention, women can navigate the challenges of stress and maintain their hormonal health.

Chapter Summary

- The adrenal glands play a crucial role in the body's stress response by releasing hormones like adrenaline and cortisol.
- Adrenaline triggers the 'fight or flight' response, increasing alertness and energy. At the same time, cortisol maintains energy supply and suppresses nonessential functions during prolonged stress.
- Chronic stress can lead to sustained high cortisol levels, causing health issues due to the body's constant alertness.
- Cortisol is essential for survival, regulating metabolism and the immune response. However, its balance is vital; chronic high levels can negatively impact women's health.
- High cortisol can disrupt sleep, cause weight gain, affect mood, and influence menstrual cycles and menopause symptoms in women.
- The concept of "adrenal fatigue" is controversial, with symptoms like fatigue and sleep disturbances, but the condition lacks robust scientific evidence.
- Managing stress is vital for hormonal balance, with strategies including a healthy diet, regular exercise, mindfulness practices, adequate sleep, and social support.
- Chronic stress can disrupt female hormonal balance, affecting menstrual cycles and fertility and increasing the risk of hormonal disorders like insulin resistance and thyroid dysfunction.

7

WEIGHT, METABOLISM, AND HORMONES

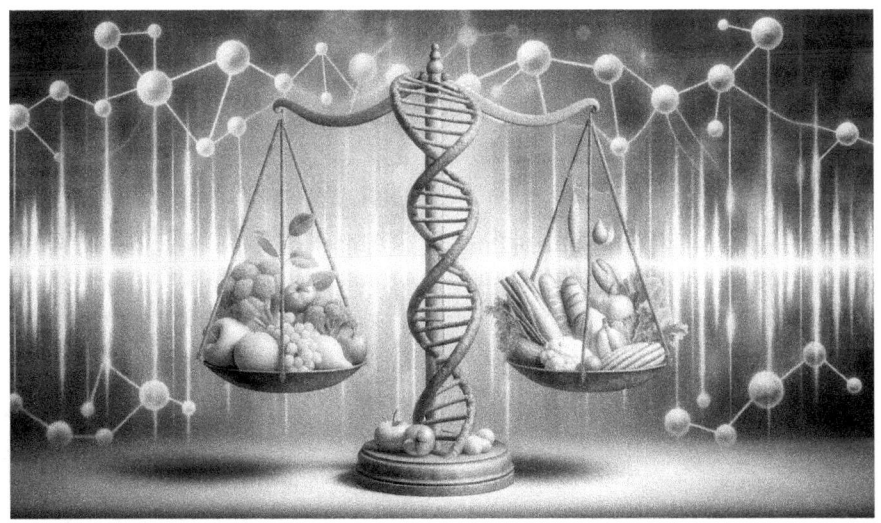

Understanding the intricate dance of hormones in your body can be like peering into a complex, ever-changing ballet. Each hormone has its role, entrance, and exit, contributing to the grand performance of your health. When it comes to weight, metabolism, and the overall energy economy of your body, hormones are the conductors, orchestrating a symphony of biological processes that can either harmonize with your health goals or, at times, seem to work against them.

One of the key players in this performance is insulin, a hormone produced by the pancreas that helps regulate blood sugar levels by facilitating glucose transport into cells for energy. Your blood sugar levels rise when you eat, signaling the pancreas to release insulin. Like a key unlocking a door, insulin allows glucose to enter the cells. As a result, your blood sugar levels begin to normalize.

However, for various reasons, sometimes the cells in your body stop responding to insulin as effectively as they should, a condition known as insulin resistance. When this happens, your pancreas works overtime, producing more insulin to get glucose into the cells. This excess insulin can have several effects on your body, including weight gain. Insulin is also known as a "storage hormone," as it signals to your body to store fat, particularly in the abdominal area, which can be especially frustrating for those trying to manage their weight.

Moreover, the relationship between insulin and weight is bidirectional. Excess body fat, particularly in the abdominal area, can increase substances known as free fatty acids, which may further promote insulin resistance. This creates a challenging cycle where weight gain can lead to more insulin resistance, which can lead to more weight gain.

But why does this happen more to some individuals than others? Genetics, lifestyle, diet, and stress levels can influence your body's sensitivity to insulin. For women, hormonal fluctuations throughout life stages, such as puberty, pregnancy, and menopause, can also impact insulin sensitivity. For instance, during menopause, the decrease in estrogen levels has been linked to an increased risk of insulin resistance.

Understanding this hormonal influence on weight is helpful because it underscores the importance of a holistic approach to weight management. It's not just about calories in versus calories out; it's about the hormonal environment within your body that affects how those calories are processed and stored.

To support healthy insulin levels and sensitivity, a balanced diet rich in fiber, healthy fats, and lean proteins can be beneficial. Regular physical activity is also key, as it can help improve insulin sensitivity by encouraging your muscles to use glucose more effectively. Additionally, managing stress and ensuring adequate sleep are important factors, as stress and sleep deprivation can negatively impact insulin sensitivity.

Remember, your body is a complex and dynamic system. While it might feel like a struggle to understand and manage the hormonal influences on your weight, know that each positive step you take is a note in the right direction, contributing to the harmony of your overall health.

Insulin Resistance and Its Impact on Health

As we delve deeper into the intricate relationship between weight, metabolism, and hormones, it's essential to understand the role of insulin resistance and its profound impact on women's health. Insulin, a hormone produced by the pancreas, is vital in managing our body's energy use. It helps cells absorb glucose from the bloodstream for energy or storage for future use. However, when insulin resistance occurs, this process becomes less efficient, and it can lead to a cascade of health issues.

Insulin resistance happens when the body's cells become less responsive to insulin. This means that despite the presence of insulin in the bloodstream, glucose remains outside the cells, leading to elevated blood sugar levels. Sensing high blood sugar, the pancreas produces even more insulin to elicit the proper cellular response. This excess insulin can create a hormonal imbalance, contributing to weight gain and difficulty losing weight.

For many women, insulin resistance is a silent condition, often going unnoticed until it manifests as prediabetes or type 2 diabetes. However, its effects on metabolism and weight can be felt long before such diagnoses. Women with insulin resistance may experience fatigue, cravings for carbohydrates, and difficulty managing their weight despite a healthy diet and exercise.

Various factors, including genetics, lifestyle choices, and hormonal changes, can influence the development of insulin resistance. Women, in particular, may face unique challenges due to hormonal fluctuations during their menstrual cycle, pregnancy, and menopause, which can all affect insulin sensitivity.

Moreover, insulin resistance is closely linked to a condition known as polycystic ovary syndrome (PCOS), which affects hormonal balance and can lead to irregular menstrual cycles, fertility issues, and weight gain. Women with PCOS often struggle with insulin resistance, which exacerbates the syndrome's symptoms and complicates its management.

Addressing insulin resistance involves a multifaceted approach. Lifestyle modifications, such as incorporating regular physical activity and adopting a balanced diet rich in fiber and low in refined sugars, can significantly improve insulin sensitivity. Sometimes, healthcare providers may recommend medication to help manage blood sugar levels.

Understanding insulin resistance is a critical step in taking control of one's hormonal health. By recognizing the signs and knowing the strategies to combat it, you can work towards restoring balance and enhancing their overall well-being. As we explore the hormonal landscape, we'll discover that hormones like leptin and ghrelin also play pivotal roles in hunger and satiety, further influencing weight and metabolism. By considering the full spectrum of hormonal interactions, we can better appreciate the complexity and interconnectedness of our body's systems.

Leptin and Ghrelin: Hunger Hormones Explained

In the intricate dance of weight management and metabolism, two key players often don't get the spotlight they deserve: leptin and ghrelin. These hormones play crucial roles in regulating hunger and satiety, acting as the body's natural messengers for when to eat and when to stop. Understanding how they work can offer us valuable insights into our relationship with food and our journey towards hormonal balance.

Leptin, often called the "satiety hormone," is produced by your fat cells. It communicates with the hypothalamus in your brain, which is the command center for appetite regulation. When you have sufficient fat stores, leptin levels increase, signaling to your brain that you have enough energy, which helps to curb your appetite. Conversely, when fat stores are low, leptin levels drop, and the brain interprets this as a sign to seek out food.

However, the story of leptin isn't always straightforward. Sometimes, despite adequate or even excessive fat stores, the brain can become less sensitive to leptin—a condition known as leptin resistance. This can lead to a perpetual feeling of hunger and overeating, as the brain doesn't receive the proper signal to stop eating. Leptin resistance is a complex issue, influenced by factors such as inflammation, high levels of fatty acids in the bloodstream, and high leptin levels itself.

On the flip side of the coin is ghrelin, the "hunger hormone," primarily produced in the stomach. Ghrelin levels rise when the stomach is empty and fall after it's filled. This hormone signals the brain that it's time to seek nourishment. If you've ever experienced those intense hunger pangs after skipping a meal, you can thank ghrelin for that urgent nudge to refuel.

The interplay between leptin and ghrelin is a delicate balance that affects not only our hunger levels but also our overall metabolic health. Disruptions in this balance can lead to weight gain and difficulty losing weight and affect energy levels and mood.

It's important to note that factors such as sleep deprivation, stress, and diet can influence the levels of these hormones. For instance, lack of sleep has been shown to decrease leptin levels and increase ghrelin, which might explain why we often feel hungrier after a poor night's sleep. Stress, too, can elevate ghrelin levels, leading to increased appetite and cravings, particularly for high-calorie comfort foods.

Understanding the roles of leptin and ghrelin can empower us to make more informed choices about our diet and lifestyle. Simple practices like getting adequate sleep, managing stress, and eating a balanced diet rich in fiber, protein, and healthy fats can help maintain the delicate balance of these hormones. Moreover, regular physical activity can improve the body's sensitivity to leptin, making it a key component in managing hunger and maintaining a healthy weight.

As we navigate the complexities of hormone health, it's clear that these hunger hormones are pivotal in the conversation about weight and metabolism. By tuning into the signals of leptin and ghrelin, we can foster a more harmonious relationship with food and support our bodies in achieving hormonal equilibrium.

The Thyroid-Weight Connection

Understanding the intricate dance between your thyroid and weight can be a revelation, especially if you've struggled with the scales despite your best efforts. The thyroid gland, a butterfly-shaped organ nestled in the front of your neck, is critical in regulating your metabolism. As we learned in earlier chapters, the thyroid produces hormones—chiefly thyroxine (T4) and triiodothyronine (T3)—that control the speed at which your body converts food into energy.

When your thyroid functions optimally, it maintains a balance that allows your metabolism to run smoothly. However, if the thyroid produces too much hormone, a condition known as hyperthyroidism, your metabolism accelerates. This can lead to weight loss, among other symptoms, but it's not a healthy or sustainable way to manage weight.

On the flip side, if your thyroid doesn't produce enough hormone—a condition called hypothyroidism—your metabolism slows down. This can lead to weight gain, and it can be frustrating because it often feels like no matter how little you eat or how much you exercise, the weight just doesn't come off.

It's essential to recognize that weight changes can be one of the first signs that your thyroid isn't functioning as it should. Women, in particular, are more susceptible to thyroid disorders, especially after pregnancy and during menopause. If you're experiencing unexpected changes in your weight, it's worth discussing with your healthcare provider whether a thyroid function test is appropriate.

Managing thyroid-related weight issues is not solely about diet and exercise; it's about getting to the root of the hormonal imbalance. If you are diagnosed with a thyroid condition, treatment typically involves hormone replacement therapy for hypothyroidism or medication to suppress hormone production for hyperthyroidism. Once your thyroid hormone levels are stabilized, your metabolism should return to a more normal rate, making managing your weight easier.

Remember, the goal is not just to reach a certain number on the scale, but to foster a healthy and balanced body. Patience is key, as it can take time for your body to adjust to new thyroid hormone levels. In the meantime, focusing on a nutrient-rich diet and regular physical activity can support overall well-being and complement any medical treatments for your thyroid.

As we move forward, we'll explore how you can proactively manage your weight by understanding and working with your body's hormonal cues. Adopting hormonal strategies for weight management can create a personalized approach that supports your body's unique needs and helps you maintain a healthy weight and metabolism.

Hormonal Strategies for Weight Management

Understanding the intricate dance of hormones and their impact on weight can be both empowering and daunting. As we've explored the significance of thyroid function in weight regulation, let's now broaden our perspective to recap some additional hormonal strategies that can aid in weight management.

Firstly, it's essential to recognize that weight management is not solely about the calories in versus calories out equation. Hormones are crucial in how your body stores fat, manages hunger and dictates energy levels. Therefore, a holistic approach to weight management should include strategies that consider hormonal balance.

One of the key players in this balance is insulin, a hormone produced by the pancreas that helps regulate blood sugar levels. When we consume foods, particularly those high in carbohydrates, our bodies break them down into glucose, which enters the bloodstream. Insulin is then released to help cells absorb and use glucose for energy. However, when insulin levels are consistently high due to a diet high in refined sugars and carbs, the body becomes less sensitive to it, a condition known as insulin resistance. This can lead to weight gain, especially around the abdomen, and increase the risk of developing type 2 diabetes.

Consider incorporating a fiber-rich diet, healthy fats, and proteins to support insulin sensitivity. These nutrients have a more gradual effect on blood sugar, which can help maintain steady insulin levels. Regular physical activity also enhances insulin sensitivity by helping the muscles absorb glucose without needing as much insulin.

Another crucial hormone for weight management is leptin, which is produced by fat cells and signals to the brain that you have enough energy stored, reducing appetite. However, just like insulin, it's possible to develop leptin resistance, where the brain no longer receives the satiety signal effectively, leading to overeating. Getting enough sleep is vital to support healthy leptin levels, as sleep deprivation can disrupt its production. Additionally, reducing inflammation through a diet rich in antioxidants from fruits, vegetables, and omega-3 fatty acids can help maintain leptin sensitivity.

Cortisol, the stress hormone, also has a significant impact on weight. Chronic stress can lead to elevated cortisol levels, which can increase appetite and drive abdominal fat storage. Managing stress through mindfulness practices, adequate sleep, and relaxation techniques can help keep cortisol levels in check.

Lastly, the balance of estrogen and progesterone can influence weight. Estrogen dominance, a condition where there is too much estrogen relative to progesterone, can lead to weight gain. To support hormonal balance, consider lifestyle changes such as reducing exposure to xenoestrogens found in plastics and certain personal care products and incorporating foods that support liver health and detoxification, like cruciferous vegetables.

In conclusion, a comprehensive approach to weight management should include dietary and exercise considerations and an understanding of how to support and balance hormones. You can create a more effective and sustainable weight management strategy that aligns with your body's natural processes by considering things like insulin sensitivity, leptin, cortisol levels, and the balance of estrogen and progesterone. Everyone's hormonal landscape is unique, so it's important to work with a healthcare provider to tailor these strategies to your needs.

Chapter Summary

- Hormones play a crucial role in weight management, metabolism, and energy regulation, with insulin being a critical hormone facilitating glucose transport into cells.
- Insulin resistance can lead to weight gain, especially abdominal fat, and is influenced by genetics, lifestyle, diet, and stress, with women experiencing additional fluctuations during life stages.
- A holistic approach to weight management should consider the hormonal environment, with a balanced diet and regular exercise improving insulin sensitivity.
- Insulin resistance is a silent condition that can lead to prediabetes or type 2 diabetes, with women facing unique challenges due to hormonal changes.
- Leptin and ghrelin are hormones that regulate hunger and satiety, with imbalances contributing to weight gain and metabolic issues.
- Sleep, stress, and diet impact leptin and ghrelin levels, affecting hunger and the ability to maintain a healthy weight.
- Thyroid hormones control metabolism, with hyperthyroidism causing weight loss and hypothyroidism leading to weight gain, particularly affecting women.
- Hormonal strategies for weight management include supporting insulin sensitivity, maintaining healthy leptin levels, managing cortisol, and balancing estrogen and progesterone.

8
MOOD, BRAIN FUNCTION, AND HORMONES

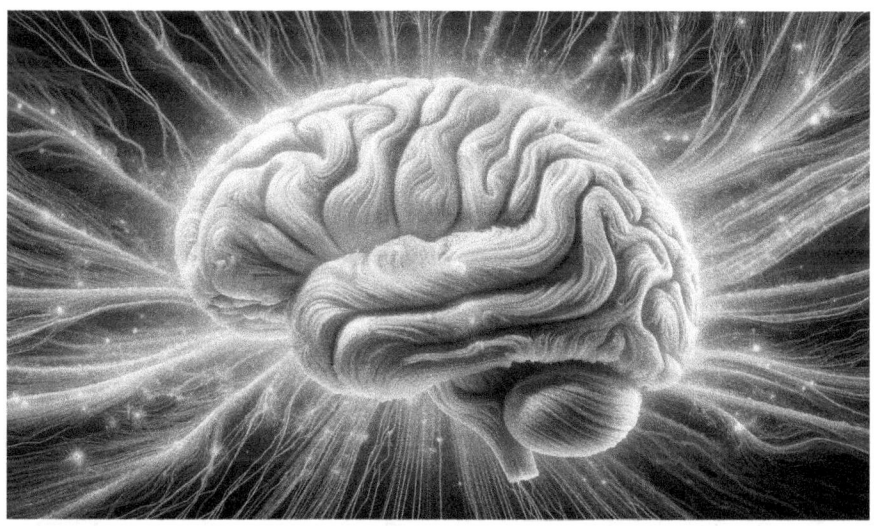

As we navigate the intricate dance of hormones within the female body, it's essential to understand their profound influence on mood. Hormones are not just chemical messengers dictating physical processes but also key players in your emotional and psychological well-being.

At the heart of this conversation is the interplay between hormones and mood. It's a complex and dynamic relationship, reflecting the ebb and flow of hormonal levels throughout life. From the onset of puberty to the transition into menopause, hormones can steer the ship of emotions, sometimes through calm waters, other times through turbulent seas.

Estrogen, one of the primary female sex hormones, has a particularly significant role in modulating mood. Fluctuations in estrogen levels can change the brain's chemistry, influencing the production and function of neurotransmitters such as serotonin, dopamine, and norepinephrine. These neurotransmitters are pivotal in regulating mood, and their balance is crucial for emotional stability.

During certain times in the menstrual cycle, particularly in the days leading up to menstruation, estrogen levels decline. Many women may experience premenstrual syndrome (PMS), which can include mood swings, irritability, and feelings of sadness. For some, these symptoms are mild and manageable. Still, for others, they can be severe and disruptive, a condition known as premenstrual dysphoric disorder (PMDD).

Pregnancy is another period of hormonal roller coaster, with estrogen and progesterone levels rising significantly. While some women feel an enhanced sense of well-being and a positive shift in mood during pregnancy, others may struggle with mood swings and even prenatal depression.

The transition to menopause, characterized by a more pronounced fluctuation and eventual decline in estrogen, can also be a time of emotional upheaval for many women. The perimenopausal period may bring about mood swings, anxiety, and depression, symptoms that can be distressing and often misunderstood.

It's not just the fluctuations that impact mood but also the brain's sensitivity to these hormonal changes. Some women may be more sensitive to shifts in estrogen and can experience more pronounced mood disturbances as a result. This sensitivity is not a sign of weakness but a reflection of the unique interplay between hormones and brain chemistry.

Understanding the hormonal underpinnings of mood is not about pathologizing the natural cycles of the female body. Instead, it's about recognizing the legitimacy of these experiences and the importance of addressing them with compassion and care. Whether through lifestyle modifications, therapeutic interventions, or medical treatments, there are many pathways to support hormone health and mood stability.

As we continue to explore the realm of female hormone health, it's clear that the mind and body are inextricably linked. The next step in our journey delves deeper into the cognitive aspects of hormonal influence, particularly how estrogen plays a role in cognitive function, memory, and overall brain health. By understanding these connections, we can better support each other in achieving physical well-being and mental and emotional harmony.

Estrogen and Cognitive Function

As we delve deeper into the intricate relationship between hormones and the female brain, it's essential to understand the role of estrogen in cognitive function. Estrogen, an essential hormone in women's health, is not only pivotal for reproductive functions but also plays a significant role in the brain's health and operation.

Estrogen's influence on cognition is multifaceted. It has been shown to have a protective effect on the brain, helping to maintain cognitive functions such as memory, attention, and problem-solving skills. This hormone interacts with neurotransmitters, the brain's chemical messengers, to enhance synaptic connectivity. It helps brain cells communicate more effectively, which is crucial for maintaining mental sharpness.

Research suggests that when estrogen levels are higher, such as the first two weeks of the menstrual cycle, some women may experience a boost in mental agility and verbal fluency. Conversely, during the latter half of the cycle, as estrogen levels decline, some may notice a slight dip in these cognitive areas. This ebb and flow is natural, but awareness can help women anticipate and understand changes in their cognitive performance throughout the month.

The impact of estrogen on the brain becomes particularly evident as women approach menopause. During this transition, the decline in estrogen can be associated with memory challenges and a decrease in the speed of cognitive processing. Some women report feelings of mental 'fogginess' during this time, which can be disconcerting. However, it's essential to recognize that this is a shared experience. Some strategies can help mitigate these effects, such as engaging in regular physical and mental exercise, maintaining a balanced diet, and, in some cases, considering hormone replacement therapy under the guidance of a healthcare professional.

Moreover, estrogen's role in brain health extends beyond cognition to mood regulation. While the previous section explored the broader impact of hormones on mood, it's worth noting that estrogen can influence the production and metabolism of neurotransmitters like serotonin and dopamine, which are directly related to mood and emotional well-being. This intricate dance between estrogen and brain chemicals is a crucial factor in understanding why some women may be more susceptible to mood swings or depression at certain times in their hormonal cycles.

Understanding estrogen's role in cognitive function is empowering. It allows you to better navigate the changes that occur throughout your life, from the menstrual cycle to menopause, and to seek support and strategies that can help maintain cognitive health and overall well-being. As we continue to explore the hormonal influences on the brain, we'll examine the connection between serotonin and premenstrual syndrome (PMS), shedding light on how hormonal fluctuations can affect emotional states in more detail.

The Serotonin Connection and PMS

As we delve into the intricate relationship between hormones and mood, it's essential to understand the role of serotonin. This critical neurotransmitter significantly influences our emotional state. For many women, the days leading up to menstruation can be marked by a cluster of physical and emotional symptoms known as premenstrual syndrome (PMS).

While PMS can manifest in various ways, mood-related symptoms such as irritability, anxiety, and sadness are among the most common. They can be profoundly disruptive to a woman's daily life.

Serotonin is often called the "feel-good" neurotransmitter because it boosts mood and creates a sense of calm. It helps regulate mood, sleep, appetite, and cognition. The connection between serotonin levels and PMS symptoms is a critical piece of the puzzle when it comes to understanding how hormonal fluctuations can affect brain function and mood.

During the menstrual cycle, levels of estrogen and progesterone rise and fall. Estrogen has a modulatory effect on serotonin receptors. As such, fluctuations in estrogen levels can lead to changes in serotonin activity. In the luteal phase of the menstrual cycle, which occurs after ovulation and before menstruation begins, estrogen levels decline. This decrease can result in reduced serotonin activity, which may contribute to mood swings and other emotional symptoms associated with PMS.

Some women may be more sensitive to these hormonal changes than others, which can explain why PMS symptoms vary widely in both type and intensity. It's also worth noting that serotonin is synthesized from tryptophan, an amino acid obtained from our diet. Nutritional factors, therefore, can also play a role in serotonin levels and, by extension, PMS symptoms.

Understanding the serotonin connection to PMS offers avenues for managing the emotional symptoms. Lifestyle modifications, such as regular exercise and a balanced diet rich in tryptophan-containing foods, can help maintain stable serotonin levels. In some cases, healthcare providers may also recommend pharmacological interventions, such as selective serotonin reuptake inhibitors (SSRIs), a class of medications that can help increase serotonin activity in the brain.

It's important to approach the management of PMS with a holistic perspective, considering the biological underpinnings and the personal and emotional experiences of each individual. By acknowledging the complex interactions between hormones, brain function, and mood, we can better support women in navigating these monthly changes with greater understanding and compassion.

As we continue to explore the impact of hormones on mental health, it becomes clear that the conversation extends beyond PMS. Hormonal influences are far-reaching, potentially affecting a range of mental health disorders. By building on our knowledge of how hormones like estrogen and neurotransmitters like serotonin interact, we can deepen our understanding of mental health and work towards more effective strategies for maintaining hormonal balance and emotional well-being.

Hormones and Mental Health Disorders

In the intricate dance of hormones and mental well-being, it's essential to recognize the profound impact that hormonal fluctuations can have on mental health disorders in women. While the previous discussion highlighted the role of serotonin, a key neurotransmitter, in premenstrual syndrome (PMS), it's important to delve deeper into the broader spectrum of mental health conditions that are influenced by hormonal changes.

Hormones such as estrogen and progesterone do more than just regulate the menstrual cycle; they also play critical roles in the brain, affecting mood, cognition, and mental health. Estrogen, for example, has a protective effect on the brain and is thought to enhance mood and cognitive function. It interacts with neurotransmitters implicated in mood disorders, such as serotonin and dopamine. This is why some women may experience mood swings, depression, or anxiety in relation to their menstrual cycle, during the postpartum period, or as they transition into menopause.

Progesterone, on the other hand, has a calming effect on the brain. It is a neurosteroid that can be a natural tranquilizer, promoting sleep and relaxation. However, the sudden drop in progesterone just before menstruation or the fluctuating levels during perimenopause can contribute to mood disturbances and anxiety.

The relationship between hormones and mental health disorders becomes even more apparent when considering conditions such as premenstrual dysphoric disorder (PMDD) and perimenopausal depression. PMDD is a severe form of PMS that can significantly disrupt a woman's life, with symptoms including intense mood swings, irritability, and depression. Perimenopausal depression, on the other hand, can emerge during the menopausal transition, a time when the hormonal landscape is changing dramatically.

Moreover, thyroid hormones also play a pivotal role in mental health. Both hyperthyroidism and hypothyroidism can manifest with symptoms that mimic mental health disorders, such as anxiety and depression. Therefore, healthcare providers must consider thyroid function when evaluating a woman presenting with mental health concerns.

It's also worth noting that hormonal contraceptives, which are widely used by women, can influence mental health. While they can stabilize hormonal fluctuations and potentially improve mood and anxiety for some, others may experience negative mood changes as a side effect. The impact of hormonal contraceptives on mental health is highly individual and emphasizes the need for personalized medical care.

Understanding the interplay between hormones and mental health is a complex yet vital part of women's health. It requires a compassionate approach that acknowledges the unique experiences of each woman. By considering the hormonal underpinnings of mental health disorders, we can pave the way for more effective, tailored treatments that address not only the psychological but also the physiological contributors to a woman's mental well-being.

As we progress, we must consider how lifestyle choices and interventions can support hormonal balance and mood regulation. Simple yet powerful lifestyle changes can often complement medical treatments, empowering women to take an active role in managing their hormonal health.

Lifestyle Choices for Hormonal Mood Regulation

In the intricate dance of hormones and emotions, knowing we are not just passive participants is empowering. Our lifestyle choices can play a pivotal role in harmonizing this delicate balance, particularly when it comes to mood regulation.

Diet, for instance, is a cornerstone of hormonal health. Foods rich in omega-3 fatty acids, such as salmon and flaxseeds, have been shown to support brain function and may help stabilize mood. Complex carbohydrates, found in whole grains and legumes, can aid in regulating blood sugar levels, which in turn can influence hormonal balance and mood. Meanwhile, limiting sugar and refined carbs is wise, which can cause spikes and dips in blood sugar and energy levels, potentially disrupting hormonal equilibrium and emotional stability.

Physical activity is another powerful tool. Regular exercise, especially aerobic activities like walking, swimming, or cycling, encourages the release of endorphins, often referred to as the body's natural mood lifters. Exercise can also help regulate the stress hormone cortisol, which, when chronically elevated, can interfere with other hormone functions.

Sleep cannot be overstated in its importance. Quality sleep is critical for the body to repair and regulate hormone production. Disrupted sleep patterns can lead to hormonal imbalances such as estrogen and progesterone, critical players in mood regulation. Establishing a calming bedtime routine and striving for 7-9 hours of sleep per night can significantly affect hormonal health.

Stress management techniques can also be beneficial, such as mindfulness meditation, yoga, or deep-breathing exercises. Chronic stress can wreak havoc on our hormonal balance, influencing cortisol levels and other hormones that affect mood. Incorporating stress-reduction practices into our daily lives can help maintain hormonal harmony and emotional well-being.

Lastly, social connections and support networks are vital. Engaging with friends, family, or support groups can provide emotional comfort and stress relief. Positive social interactions can trigger the release of oxytocin, a hormone that promotes feelings of bonding and reduces stress responses.

Integrating these lifestyle interventions can support our hormonal health and foster a more stable mood landscape. It's a proactive approach that enhances our emotional well-being and empowers us to take charge of our overall health. Remember, small, consistent changes can lead to significant improvements over time, and it's never too late to start nurturing your hormonal harmony.

Chapter Summary

- Hormones, particularly estrogen, play a significant role in women's mood regulation, influencing neurotransmitters like serotonin, dopamine, and norepinephrine.
- Fluctuations in estrogen levels can cause mood swings and conditions like premenstrual syndrome (PMS) and premenstrual dysphoric disorder (PMDD), especially before menstruation.
- Pregnancy and menopause are periods of hormonal changes that can significantly affect a woman's mood, with some experiencing mood swings, anxiety, and depression.
- Individual sensitivity to hormonal changes can lead to varying degrees of mood disturbances among women.
- Estrogen is also crucial for cognitive functions such as memory and attention, with its levels affecting mental agility and verbal fluency.
- The serotonin connection to PMS highlights the role of diet and lifestyle in managing mood-related symptoms, with options like exercise, balanced diet, and SSRIs as treatments.
- Hormonal fluctuations can impact mental health disorders beyond PMS, with estrogen and progesterone affecting mood and cognition and thyroid hormones influencing mental health.
- Lifestyle choices, including diet, exercise, sleep, stress management, and social connections, can significantly influence hormonal balance and mood regulation.

9

SKIN, HAIR, AND HORMONES

When we think of our skin, we often consider it merely as a protective barrier or an aesthetic feature. However, it's much more than that—it's a complex organ intimately connected with our internal processes, including hormones. Understanding this connection can be particularly enlightening for women, as hormonal fluctuations throughout life stages can manifest visibly on the skin.

Hormones play a significant role in the health and appearance of our skin. Estrogen and progesterone, the primary female sex hormones, influence skin thickness, wrinkle formation, and moisture. They can enhance collagen production, giving skin its youthful, supple structure. Conversely, when these hormone levels decline, such as during menopause, the skin may lose elasticity and become drier.

Testosterone, though typically considered a male hormone, is present in women as well and can have a profound impact on the skin. Excess testosterone can increase sebum production, the oily substance that can clog pores and lead to acne. This is why some women experience breakouts not just during puberty, when hormone levels fluctuate dramatically, but also at specific points in their menstrual cycle, during pregnancy, or in conditions like polycystic ovary syndrome (PCOS), where testosterone levels may be elevated.

The thyroid hormones produced by the thyroid gland also play a crucial role in skin health. They help regulate skin cell renewal. When the thyroid is overactive (hyperthyroidism) or underactive (hypothyroidism), it can lead to a variety of skin issues. Hyperthyroidism may cause warm, moist, and smooth skin, while hypothyroidism can lead to dry, rough, and cold skin.

Cortisol, the stress hormone, can also affect the skin. Chronic stress leads to prolonged cortisol elevation, which can break down collagen and elastin, the fibers that give skin firmness and elasticity. This can accelerate aging, leading to the earlier onset of wrinkles and sagging skin.

It's not just the presence of these hormones that matters, but their balance. Hormonal imbalances can lead to various skin conditions, from dryness and sensitivity to acne and hirsutism (excessive hair growth). It's a delicate dance that changes with the rhythms of life—puberty, the menstrual cycle, pregnancy, and menopause.

Understanding the skin-hormone connection is empowering. It allows women to anticipate changes in their skin and seek appropriate treatments. Lifestyle choices, such as diet, exercise, and stress management, can influence hormone levels and, by extension, skin health. Additionally, topical treatments, medications, and hormone replacement therapies can be tailored to address specific skin concerns related to hormonal changes.

Our skin reflects our inner health, including the complex symphony of hormones that play throughout a woman's life. By nurturing our hormonal health, we also care for our skin, ensuring it remains as resilient and vibrant as possible.

Acne and Hormones: Beyond the Teenage Years

As we gracefully navigate beyond the tumultuous seas of teenage years, many of us anticipate leaving particular unwelcome companions at the shore, acne being a prime candidate. Yet, for numerous women, the reality is that acne can persist or even first appear in adulthood, often leaving them perplexed and seeking answers.

Understanding the intricate dance of hormones within our bodies is crucial in unraveling the mystery of adult acne. While adolescence is notorious for hormonal upheavals, the truth is that our endocrine system continues to ebb and flow throughout our lives, influenced by factors such as the menstrual cycle, pregnancy, birth control, and the approach of menopause.

Androgens, a group of hormones that includes testosterone, often play the lead role in the story of adult acne. These hormones can cause the sebaceous glands in the skin to produce more oil, which can lead to clogged pores and the proliferation of acne-causing bacteria. For women, fluctuations in androgen levels can be particularly pronounced during certain times of the menstrual cycle, as well as in conditions such as polycystic ovary syndrome (PCOS), where androgen levels are typically higher.

But it's not just about androgens. Estrogen and progesterone also influence skin health, with estrogen known for its skin-friendly properties, such as promoting collagen production and improving skin elasticity. As these hormone levels fluctuate, so too can the clarity and overall condition of the skin.

Stress, too, can be a significant factor. It triggers the release of cortisol, a hormone that can indirectly increase androgen levels and exacerbate skin issues. This is why, during periods of high stress, you might notice a sudden flare-up of acne, even if you're well past your teenage years.

Treatment for hormonal acne in adulthood often involves a multifaceted approach. Topical treatments and good skincare habits are the first line of defense, but for many, addressing the hormonal root of the issue is vital. This may involve the use of oral contraceptives, which can help regulate hormone levels or other medications that specifically target androgens.

Lifestyle changes can also be impactful. A balanced diet, regular exercise, and stress management techniques can all help regulate hormone levels and support overall skin health. Additionally, it's important to consider the role of skincare products and routines. Non-comedogenic products that don't clog pores and gentle, non-irritating ingredients can be beneficial in managing adult acne.

Navigating the complexities of hormone health requires patience and often a touch of trial and error. It's essential to remember that each individual's hormonal landscape is unique, and what works for one person may not work for another. Consulting with healthcare professionals, such as dermatologists or endocrinologists, can provide tailored advice and treatment options.

In the journey to understand and manage adult acne, it's essential to approach the situation with kindness towards oneself. The skin is not just an external organ; it reflects the intricate internal processes that make each woman unique. By addressing hormonal health holistically, it's possible to find solutions that clear the skin and support overall well-being.

Hair Loss and Excess Hair Growth: Hormonal Influences

As we navigate the complexities of our bodies, it's clear that hormones play a pivotal role in the health and appearance of our skin and hair. For many women, hair density and distribution changes can be a source of concern and confusion. Understanding the hormonal influences behind hair loss and excess hair growth can empower us to address these issues with greater insight and compassion.

Hair loss, or alopecia, can be particularly distressing. It's not just about vanity; our hair is often tied to our identity and sense of femininity. Various hormonal factors can contribute to hair thinning in women. A common culprit is androgenetic alopecia, also known as female pattern hair loss, which is influenced by androgens, including testosterone. While androgens are typically considered male hormones, they are present in all bodies. They can affect hair follicles by shortening the growth phase of the hair cycle, leading to thinner, shorter hairs.

Another hormonal condition that can lead to hair loss is thyroid dysfunction. Both hyperthyroidism (an overactive thyroid) and hypothyroidism (an underactive thyroid) can cause hair to become thin and brittle, often resulting in diffuse hair shedding. The thyroid gland plays a crucial role in regulating metabolism and energy use in the body. When it's out of balance, hair growth can be significantly impacted.

On the flip side, some women experience hirsutism, which is the growth of coarse, dark hair in areas where men typically grow hair, such as the face, chest, and back. This condition is often linked to an excess of androgens or an increased sensitivity of hair follicles to these hormones. Polycystic ovary syndrome (PCOS) is a common hormonal disorder that can cause both hirsutism and hair thinning on the scalp due to its association with elevated androgen levels.

It's important to recognize that these hair-related changes are not just cosmetic issues but can signal underlying health concerns. They can also take a toll on emotional well-being, leading to stress and anxiety, which, in a challenging cycle, can further exacerbate hair problems. Stress hormones like cortisol can disrupt the hair growth cycle, leading to telogen effluvium, a temporary condition where hair falls out after a stressful event.

Navigating these changes requires a multifaceted approach. It often involves working with healthcare providers to diagnose and treat underlying hormonal imbalances. Additionally, lifestyle modifications, such as managing stress, can play a supportive role in improving hair health.

In the journey toward hormonal balance and hair health, it's crucial to approach the subject with kindness towards oneself. The changes you are experiencing are not a reflection of your worth or beauty. By understanding the hormonal influences on hair, you can take informed steps toward managing your hair health while nurturing your overall well-being.

Natural Approaches to Hormonal Skin and Hair Health

In the intricate dance of hormones and health, our skin and hair often reflect the inner balance—or imbalance—of our body's hormonal symphony. As we've explored the hormonal influences on hair loss and excess hair growth, it's clear that hormones play a pivotal role in our skin and hair condition. But what can we do to foster hormonal harmony naturally and, in turn, enhance the health and appearance of our skin and hair?

First and foremost, it's important to acknowledge that each individual's hormonal landscape is unique, and what works for one person may not work for another. However, several natural approaches can support overall hormone health, which may positively affect your skin and hair.

One of the simplest yet most profound changes you can make is prioritizing sleep. Quality sleep is a cornerstone of hormonal balance. During sleep, our bodies repair and regenerate, including synthesizing and regulating hormones. Aim for 7-9 hours of restful sleep per night, and consider adopting a calming bedtime routine to help signal to your body that it's time to wind down.

Stress management is another key factor. Chronic stress can wreak havoc on hormone levels, particularly cortisol, the stress hormone, which can, in turn, affect skin and hair. Techniques such as deep breathing, meditation, yoga, or a leisurely walk can help manage stress levels. They may contribute to a more balanced hormonal state.

Exercise is a powerful tool for hormonal health. Regular physical activity can help regulate insulin levels, support healthy estrogen metabolism, and boost mood-enhancing endorphins. Whether it's a brisk walk, a dance class, or weight training, find a form of exercise you enjoy and make it a consistent part of your routine.

Herbal remedies and supplements may also play a supportive role. For instance, spearmint tea has been studied for its potential to reduce androgens, like testosterone, which can contribute to hormonal acne and hirsutism. Vitex (also known as chasteberry) is another herb that's traditionally been used to support female hormonal balance. However, it's crucial to consult with a healthcare provider before starting any new supplement, especially if you have a medical condition or are taking medications.

Topical natural treatments can also be beneficial for skin and hair. For example, tea tree oil has antimicrobial properties and may help acne-prone skin when diluted and applied topically. Similarly, oils like coconut or argan oil can nourish the scalp and hair, potentially improving hair texture and strength.

Lastly, consider the role of gentle detoxification. Our bodies are equipped with natural detoxification systems, but supporting these processes through hydration, a diet rich in fiber, and detoxifying foods like cruciferous vegetables can aid in eliminating excess hormones and toxins that may be affecting your skin and hair health.

Remember, the journey to hormonal balance is often gradual, and patience is vital. Small, consistent changes can lead to significant improvements over time. By embracing these natural approaches, you're nurturing your skin and hair and supporting your overall well-being.

The Impact of Diet on Skin and Hair

In our journey through understanding the intimate relationship between our hormones and the health of our skin and hair, we've explored the natural strategies that can support this delicate balance. Now, let's delve into nutrition and its profound impact on our hormonal well-being, mainly focusing on the skin and hair.

The adage "you are what you eat" holds a kernel of truth, especially regarding our skin and hair health. The foods we consume can either support or disrupt hormonal balance, which in turn can manifest in our external appearance. A diet rich in certain nutrients can help fortify the skin and hair, making them more resilient against hormonal fluctuations.

Firstly, let's consider the role of antioxidants. These powerful substances combat oxidative stress, which hormonal imbalances can exacerbate. Foods high in antioxidants, such as berries, dark leafy greens, and nuts, can help protect the skin from the premature aging that free radicals can cause. They also support the body's natural detoxification processes, which are crucial for maintaining hormonal equilibrium.

Another key player in the diet-skin-hair connection is omega-3 fatty acids. Found in abundance in fatty fish like salmon, flaxseeds, and walnuts, omega-3s are known for their anti-inflammatory properties.

Inflammation can be a response to hormonal changes, and by mitigating this response, omega-3s can help to keep skin clear and hair strong.

Protein is the building block of hair, and ensuring adequate intake is essential for hair health. Hormonal shifts can sometimes lead to hair thinning or loss, and a diet rich in high-quality protein from sources like eggs, poultry, and legumes can provide the necessary nutrients to help maintain hair strength and growth.

Furthermore, vitamins and minerals play a significant role. For instance, vitamin E in avocados and almonds can help protect the skin from damage and support its healing processes. Zinc, present in pumpkin seeds and chickpeas, is crucial for skin repair, hormone production, and regulation.

It's also important to consider the impact of certain foods and substances that might disrupt hormonal balance. High-glycemic foods, for example, can cause spikes in insulin, which may exacerbate conditions like acne. Similarly, dairy products have been linked to hormonal disturbances in some individuals. Being mindful of how these foods affect your body can guide you in making dietary choices that support your hormonal health.

Hydration, too, cannot be overstated. Water is essential for every cellular function in our bodies, including regulating hormones and maintaining skin and hair health. Ensuring adequate hydration helps to keep the skin supple and can even prevent the scalp from becoming dry and flaky.

Incorporating a balanced diet that supports hormonal health doesn't have to be a chore. It can be a delightful exploration of flavors and foods that nourish your body and bring joy and satisfaction to your meals. Remember, the journey to hormonal balance is personal, and what works for one may not work for another. It's about listening to your body, observing how it responds to different foods, and adjusting your diet.

By embracing a diet that supports hormonal balance, you're taking a proactive step towards healthier skin and hair and overall well-being. As we continue to explore the multifaceted aspects of hormone health, remember that each choice you make at the dining table can be a powerful ally in your quest for vitality and harmony within your body.

Chapter Summary

- The skin is deeply connected to hormonal processes, with hormone fluctuations like estrogen, progesterone, and testosterone affecting its health and appearance.
- Hormonal changes during life stages such as puberty, menstrual cycles, pregnancy, and menopause can visibly impact the skin, causing acne, dryness, and wrinkles.
- Testosterone can increase sebum production and lead to acne. At the same time, thyroid hormones affect skin cell renewal, with imbalances causing various skin conditions.
- Cortisol, the stress hormone, can break down skin-supporting collagen and elastin, accelerating aging and causing wrinkles and sagging skin.
- Hormonal imbalances can lead to skin conditions such as acne and hirsutism (excessive hair growth), with a balance being crucial for skin health.
- Lifestyle choices, topical treatments, medications, and hormone therapies can help manage skin concerns related to hormonal changes.
- Adult acne can persist beyond teenage years due to hormonal fluctuations, with treatment often involving a combination of skincare, medication, and lifestyle changes.
- Hair health is also influenced by hormones, with conditions like androgenetic alopecia, thyroid dysfunction affecting hair density, and hirsutism causing excess hair growth.

10
INTEGRATIVE APPROACHES TO HORMONE HEALTH

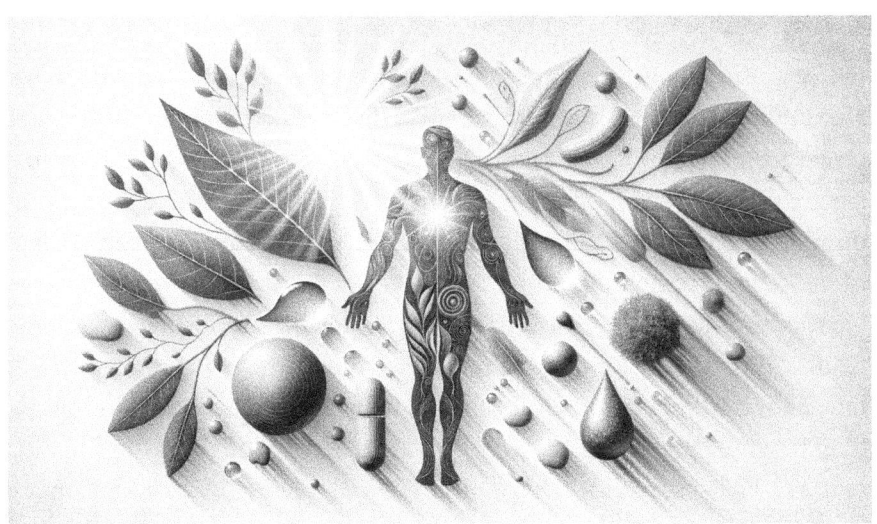

As we navigate the intricate dance of hormones within our bodies, we must recognize the profound impact our lifestyle choices have on this delicate balance.

The Role of Diet in Hormone Balance

The foods we consume can be messengers, sending signals that harmonize or disrupt our hormonal symphony.

To begin with, let's consider the building blocks of hormones: fats. Not all fats are created equal, and the quality of fats matters most. Healthy fats, such as those found in avocados, nuts, seeds, and oily fish, are necessary for hormone production and function. These fats contribute to the structural integrity of cell membranes, allowing hormones to communicate with each cell in the body effectively.

On the other hand, processed and trans fats found in many baked goods and fried foods can interfere with hormone receptors, leading to miscommunication and potential hormonal imbalances. It's like trying to have a clear conversation in a room filled with static; the message gets lost along the way.

Next, let's talk about fiber. Found in fruits, vegetables, legumes, and whole grains, fiber plays a crucial role in hormone health by aiding in the elimination of excess hormones, particularly estrogen. When estrogen levels are too high, it can lead to a variety of issues, including menstrual irregularities and mood swings. By ensuring a high-fiber diet, we support our body's natural detoxification processes, helping to maintain a harmonious hormonal environment.

Moreover, certain nutrients are pivotal in supporting hormonal health. For instance, magnesium, found in leafy greens and dark chocolate, assists in regulating cortisol, our stress hormone. B vitamins, abundant in whole grains and leafy greens, are essential for energy production and synthesizing various hormones. Vitamin D, which we can obtain from sunlight and fortified foods, is crucial for reproductive health and mood regulation.

It's also worth noting the importance of maintaining stable blood sugar levels. Frequent spikes and crashes can wreak havoc on insulin, our blood sugar-regulating hormone, and can subsequently affect other hormones such as cortisol and estrogen. To promote stable blood sugar, it's advisable to include a balanced combination of protein, healthy fats, and complex carbohydrates with each meal.

Lastly, let's not forget the role of phytoestrogens, plant-based compounds that can mimic estrogen in the body. Found in foods like soy, flaxseeds, and sesame seeds, phytoestrogens can be particularly beneficial during menopause, when the body's natural estrogen levels decline. However, the key is moderation and variety, as the effects of phytoestrogens can vary from person to person.

In summary, the foods we choose to nourish our bodies can profoundly affect our hormonal health. By focusing on whole, nutrient-dense foods and avoiding those that can disrupt hormonal communication, we lay the foundation for a balanced endocrine system. As we move forward, we'll explore how pairing these dietary choices with physical activity can enhance hormonal harmony, creating a holistic approach to health and well-being.

Exercise and Hormonal Health

In the tapestry of factors contributing to hormone health, exercise emerges as a vibrant thread, interwoven with the dietary patterns we explored earlier. Physical activity, in its many forms, profoundly impacts hormonal balance, influencing everything from stress hormones to reproductive hormones. It's a tool that, when used appropriately, can harmonize the body's endocrine symphony.

Let's begin by understanding that not all exercise is created equal in the eyes of our hormones. The type and intensity of activity can lead to different hormonal responses. For instance, moderate aerobic exercise, such as brisk walking or cycling, can boost the production of endorphins, the body's natural mood elevators. This can be particularly beneficial for women who may experience mood fluctuations associated with hormonal changes.

Resistance training, on the other hand, plays a crucial role in managing insulin sensitivity and glucose metabolism. By building lean muscle mass, women can enhance their metabolic rate, which can help regulate blood sugar levels and reduce the risk of insulin resistance—a condition that can lead to type 2 diabetes and is often associated with polycystic ovary syndrome (PCOS).

Furthermore, exercise can influence the delicate balance of estrogen and progesterone, two key players in women's reproductive health. Regular physical activity has been shown to help regulate menstrual cycles and alleviate symptoms of premenstrual syndrome (PMS) and menopause. However, it's important to note that excessive exercise or high-intensity training without adequate recovery can disrupt this balance, potentially leading to irregular periods or amenorrhea (the absence of menstruation).

Stress hormones, particularly cortisol, are also responsive to exercise. While acute bouts of exercise temporarily increase cortisol levels, chronic stress without proper rest can lead to sustained high levels of this hormone, which may disrupt overall hormonal balance. Incorporating restorative practices such as yoga or tai chi can help mitigate stress and promote a more favorable cortisol profile.

As we consider the role of exercise in hormonal health, it's essential to embrace a personalized approach. Each woman's body is unique, and what constitutes a harmonizing activity for one may not have the same effect for another. Listening to one's body and responding to its cues is paramount. This means adjusting exercise routines to align with energy levels, menstrual cycles, and life's demands.

In this journey towards hormonal equilibrium, it's also important to remember that rest is as vital as activity. Just as we need sleep to restore and rejuvenate (a topic we'll delve into more deeply in the following section), our bodies require downtime to repair and adapt to the beneficial stresses imposed by exercise.

In summary, integrating exercise into our lives is not just about pursuing fitness; it's about nurturing our hormonal health. By choosing activities that resonate with our bodies and lifestyles and balancing exertion with rest, we can use exercise as a powerful ally in achieving hormonal harmony.

Sleep's Influence on Hormonal Regulation

As we nestle into the comforting embrace of a good night's sleep, our bodies embark on an intricate dance of hormonal regulation and rebalancing. This nightly ritual is not merely about rest and recovery; it's a critical time for our endocrine system to perform essential maintenance that impacts our overall hormone health.

The relationship between sleep and hormones is a reciprocal one. Just as our hormone levels can influence how well we sleep, the quality and quantity of our sleep can profoundly affect our hormonal balance. This balance is particularly delicate and significant for women, as it governs everything from menstrual cycles to mood regulation.

One of the most well-known sleep-related hormones is melatonin, often called the "sleep hormone." Produced by the pineal gland in the brain, melatonin helps regulate our sleep-wake cycle, signaling to our bodies when it's time to wind down and prepare for sleep. Exposure to light at night can suppress melatonin production, which is why it's recommended to reduce screen time before bed to encourage a healthy sleep cycle.

But melatonin is just the beginning. Sleep also influences other hormones that are pivotal in women's health. For instance, during sleep, the body can regulate cortisol. High cortisol levels can disrupt various bodily functions, including menstrual regularity and ovulation. Women can help keep cortisol levels in check by ensuring adequate sleep and promoting a sense of calm and stability throughout the body.

Growth hormone is another key player during sleep. It helps repair and regenerate cells, supports muscle growth, and aids in the metabolism of fats. This hormone is primarily secreted during deep sleep, highlighting the importance of the duration and quality of sleep we get each night.

Furthermore, sleep impacts insulin, the hormone responsible for regulating blood sugar levels. Poor sleep can lead to insulin resistance, which can increase the risk of diabetes and weight gain. For women, particularly those with polycystic ovary syndrome (PCOS), managing insulin levels through adequate sleep is crucial for maintaining hormonal equilibrium.

Leptin and ghrelin, the hormones associated with hunger and satiety, are also influenced by our sleep patterns. A lack of sleep can lead to an increase in ghrelin, the hunger hormone, and a decrease in leptin, which signals fullness. This imbalance can result in increased cravings and a tendency to overeat, making sleep a vital component of weight management and metabolic health.

For women navigating the ebb and flow of hormonal changes throughout their lives, from menstruation to menopause, sleep becomes an essential foundation for hormonal health. It's a time for the body to reset, rebalance, and restore itself.

Establishing a consistent sleep routine is vital to harnessing the power of sleep for hormonal regulation. This includes going to bed and waking up at the same time each day, creating a restful sleep environment, and engaging in relaxing activities before bedtime. Women can support their hormonal health and enhance their overall well-being by prioritizing sleep.

As we continue exploring integrative approaches to hormone health, it becomes clear that the mind and body are interconnected. The practices that support our mental and emotional states can profoundly affect our hormonal balance. With this understanding, we can appreciate the holistic nature of our health and the various ways we can nurture it.

Mind-Body Practices for Hormonal Harmony

As we journey through the landscape of hormone health, we must recognize the profound connection between our minds and bodies. This connection is not just poetic—it's physiological. The symphony of hormones that influences everything from our mood to our metabolism is highly sensitive to our mental and emotional states. Embracing mind-body practices can be a powerful way to promote hormonal harmony.

One of the most accessible and effective mind-body practices is meditation. Meditation has been shown to reduce stress, which can help regulate cortisol levels. Cortisol can wreak havoc on other hormones when it's chronically elevated. By incorporating a daily meditation practice, even if it's just for a few minutes, you can create a space of calm within your day. This tranquility signals to your endocrine system that all is well, allowing your body to maintain a more balanced hormonal state.

Yoga, another integrative practice, combines physical postures, breath control, and meditation. It's particularly beneficial for women's hormone health because it reduces stress and supports the endocrine system through specific poses that can stimulate or soothe various glands. For instance, poses like forward folds can calm the adrenal glands, while shoulder stands may invigorate the thyroid. Yoga's holistic approach nurtures the entire body and mind, fostering an environment where hormones can flourish in balance.

Deep breathing exercises, or pranayama in the yogic tradition, are also invaluable. Deep, diaphragmatic breathing activates the parasympathetic nervous system, responsible for the 'rest and digest' state. This state is crucial for allowing the body to repair and regulate itself, including hormonal functions. By practicing deep breathing, you can help reduce the fight-or-flight response triggered by stress and encourage a more harmonious hormonal milieu.

Biofeedback is a more technologically advanced mind-body technique that can also aid in managing hormone health. It involves using electronic monitoring to convey information about physiological processes. With this feedback, you can learn to control certain bodily functions that are usually involuntary, like heart rate or muscle tension. Over time, biofeedback can teach you to mitigate your body's stress response and improve conditions like PMS or menopausal symptoms, which are often exacerbated by stress.

Lastly, mindfulness can be woven throughout your day to maintain a state of hormonal equilibrium. Mindfulness involves being fully present and engaged in the moment without judgment. This can mean savoring your food, which can help with digestive hormones, or being fully attentive during conversations, reducing stress and improving your emotional well-being.

Incorporating these mind-body practices into your life doesn't require a complete lifestyle overhaul. It's about finding moments to pause, breathe, and connect with yourself throughout your day. By doing so, you're not just nurturing your mind but taking an active role in your hormone health. As we move forward, remember that the journey to hormonal health is about what we put into our bodies and how we tune into our internal rhythms and cultivate inner peace.

Navigating Hormone Therapy and Supplements

As we delve into the realm of hormone therapy and supplements, it's essential to approach this topic with a blend of caution, curiosity, and a deep respect for the intricate symphony of your body's hormonal system. Hormone therapy and the use of supplements can be powerful tools in the quest for hormonal balance. Still, they have their complexities and potential risks.

When considering hormone therapy, it's essential to understand that this approach often involves replacing or supplementing hormones in your body to alleviate symptoms associated with hormonal imbalances or deficiencies. This can be particularly relevant during life transitions such as perimenopause and menopause or in conditions like hypothyroidism or polycystic ovary syndrome (PCOS).

However, hormone therapy is not a one-size-fits-all solution. It requires a personalized approach, often starting with comprehensive testing to determine your specific hormonal needs. Blood, saliva, or urine tests can provide a snapshot of your hormonal landscape, guiding your healthcare provider in tailoring a treatment plan for you.

When it comes to hormone replacement therapy (HRT), there are several options available, including bioidentical hormones, which are chemically identical to those your body produces naturally. These can come in various forms, such as pills, patches, creams, or gels. The decision to use bioidentical hormones should be made in collaboration with a healthcare professional who can help weigh the benefits against potential risks, such as the increased risk of certain cancers or cardiovascular events associated with some forms of HRT.

Supplements, on the other hand, can offer a more indirect approach to supporting hormone health. They can include a range of vitamins, minerals, herbs, and other nutraceuticals that may help to support the body's natural hormone production and balance. For instance, vitamin D and magnesium are crucial for bone health, especially as estrogen levels decline during menopause. Omega-3 fatty acids can support mood and reduce inflammation. At the same time, adaptogenic herbs like ashwagandha may help the body cope with stress and support adrenal health.

It's vital to approach supplements with the same level of scrutiny as any other treatment. Not all supplements are created equal, and their quality can vary widely. It's advisable to look for products that have been third-party tested for purity and potency. Furthermore, discussing any supplements you're considering with your healthcare provider is essential, as they can interact with medications and may not be appropriate for everyone.

Remember, hormone therapy and supplements are just one piece of the puzzle. They can be effective when used judiciously and in conjunction with other lifestyle interventions, such as a balanced diet, regular exercise, adequate sleep, and stress management techniques. Your body is a complex and dynamic system, and nurturing hormone health is a journey that often requires a multifaceted approach.

As you navigate the options available to you, keep in mind that your journey is unique. What works for one person may not work for another. It's about finding harmony within your body and working with healthcare professionals who listen to you, understand your goals, and help you make informed decisions about your hormone health. With patience and persistence, you can find a path that addresses your symptoms and enhances your overall well-being.

Chapter Summary

- Dietary choices significantly influence hormonal balance, with certain foods acting as messengers that can harmonize or disrupt the endocrine system.
- Healthy fats are essential for hormone production and function, while processed and trans fats can interfere with hormone receptors.
- Fiber aids in eliminating excess hormones, particularly estrogen, and supports the body's natural detoxification processes.
- Nutrients like magnesium, B vitamins, and Vitamin D are pivotal for regulating stress hormones, energy production, and reproductive health.
- Maintaining stable blood sugar levels is crucial for hormonal balance, and a diet balanced with protein, fats, and complex carbs can help.
- Phytoestrogens found in foods like soy and flaxseeds can mimic estrogen in the body and are beneficial in moderation, especially during menopause.
- Exercise impacts hormonal health, with different types and intensities of activity influencing stress and reproductive hormones.
- Adequate sleep is critical for hormonal regulation, affecting hormones like melatonin, cortisol, growth hormone, insulin, leptin, and ghrelin.

YOUR HORMONAL JOURNEY

As we conclude this book, it's time to reflect on our journey together. We've navigated the complex landscape of the endocrine system, uncovering how hormones influence every aspect of a woman's health. From the onset of puberty to the transition to menopause, we've explored the pivotal moments that define the hormonal experience of womanhood.

This journey has revealed the delicate balance hormones bring to our lives, impacting our physical well-being, emotional states, and mental clarity. We've learned that small messengers can have powerful effects and that understanding their language is vital to maintaining our health. The knowledge gained here serves as a foundation for building a more attuned relationship with your body.

We've also seen that hormonal imbalances are not destinies set in stone but are challenges that can be met with informed strategies and compassionate self-care. Recognizing the signs of imbalance and responding with appropriate interventions can steer your health toward equilibrium.

The journey continues after the last page of this book. It's an ongoing process of listening to your body, adapting to its needs, and advocating for your well-being. As you continue to grow and change, so will your hormonal needs. With the insights and tools you've acquired, you're better prepared to face those changes confidently and gracefully. Remember, your hormonal health is a personal voyage that you navigate with the wisdom and understanding you've gathered along the way.

Celebrating Empowerment and Self-Care

The voyage through this book has been one of discovery and empowerment. By delving into the intricacies of the endocrine system and its profound impact on every facet of your life, you've taken an important step towards self-care and personal well-being. This book has aimed to arm you with the knowledge to become an advocate for your health, understanding that hormonal balance is a cornerstone of your overall vitality.

Empowerment comes from recognizing that you have the tools and information to influence your hormonal health positively. You've learned about the importance of diet, exercise, stress management, and sleep—each a powerful lever in your control. By making conscious choices in these areas, you can support your endocrine system and enhance your quality of life.

Self-care is an act of self-love, and by prioritizing it, you honor your body's needs. The practices and insights shared in this book encourage you to listen to your body's signals and respond with nurturing actions. Whether through a nourishing meal, a rejuvenating workout, or a moment of mindfulness, each act of self-care is a celebration of your commitment to your health.

As you continue on your path, remember that self-care is not a destination but a journey that requires patience, kindness, and perseverance. Celebrate each step you take and each choice you make in favor of your well-being. The empowerment you've gained through this journey is a testament to your strength and dedication to living a balanced and healthy life.

The Future of Your Hormonal Health

As you close the final chapter, it's essential to look forward to the future of your hormonal health with optimism and a proactive mindset. The journey to understanding and managing your hormones is an evolving process that will continue to unfold as you move through life's stages and face new challenges.

The field of hormone health is dynamic, with ongoing research and advancements that promise to deepen our understanding and improve our approaches to care. Staying abreast of these developments is crucial, as they may offer new insights into treatments, therapies, and preventative measures that can further enhance your well-being.

Your hormonal health journey is also subject to change. Your hormonal needs will evolve as your body ages and your life circumstances shift. This book has equipped you with a solid foundation, but it's essential to remain vigilant and responsive to your body's cues. Regular check-ups with healthcare professionals, staying informed about your options, and making lifestyle adjustments as necessary are all part of maintaining hormonal balance over time.

Embrace the future with the knowledge that you are not a passive participant in your hormonal health. You have the power to influence it through the choices you make every day. Whether through nutrition, exercise, stress management, or medical intervention, you have the tools to support your endocrine system and thrive. The future of your hormonal health is bright, and with the wisdom you've gained, you're well-prepared to meet it head-on.

Continue Learning and Growing

The conclusion of this book is not an end but a call to action—a beckoning towards continued learning and growth in your hormonal health journey. The empowerment you've gained through understanding your hormones and endocrine system is just the beginning. It's a foundation upon which you can build a lifetime of well-being, adapting to the ever-changing landscape of your body's needs.

I urge you to remain curious and proactive. Seek out new information, stay updated with the latest research, and consider how emerging science can benefit your personal health narrative. Your body is a living library of signals and symptoms; learning to read and interpret these cues is a skill that will serve you well throughout your life.

Engage with communities that share your commitment to hormonal health. Whether through online forums, local support groups, or wellness workshops, connecting with others provides a wealth of shared knowledge and mutual encouragement. These networks can be invaluable resources as you navigate the complexities of hormonal balance.

Remember, your journey is unique; what works for one may not work for another. Be willing to experiment, to listen to your body, and to adjust your approach as necessary. Your path to hormonal harmony is one of personal evolution, requiring patience, resilience, and an open mind.

Take this call to action to heart. Continue to learn, to grow, and to thrive. Your health is a lifelong quest, and with each step, you grow stronger and more attuned to your body's needs. Embrace this journey with confidence and the knowledge that you can cultivate the vibrant health you deserve.

Nurturing Your Hormonal Balance Beyond the Pages

As we part ways, I extend to you heartfelt words of support and encouragement. This book has been a vessel of knowledge, a guide through the sometimes turbulent waters of hormonal health, but the journey doesn't end here. It continues with each day you commit to understanding and nurturing your body.

Remember, you are not alone on this path. Countless women are on similar journeys, each with a story of challenges and triumphs. Draw strength from this collective experience and know your efforts to achieve hormonal balance are important and shared.

Take pride in the steps you've already taken. Whether minor adjustments or significant changes, each one is a victory in its own right. Celebrate your progress and be gentle with yourself when faced with setbacks. Hormonal health is not about perfection; it's about striving for balance and well-being within the beautiful complexity of your body.

I encourage you to hold onto the hope and determination that have brought you this far. Continue to advocate for your health with the wisdom and tools you've acquired. Your journey is one of empowerment, a testament to your resilience and dedication to living your best life.

As you move forward, carry with you the knowledge that you are capable, strong, and fully equipped to navigate the ever-changing landscape of your hormonal health. May this book remain a trusted friend, and you step into the future with confidence and grace. Your path to hormonal harmony is yours to shape, and I am cheering for you at every step.

ABOUT THE AUTHOR

Lila Lacy is a passionate advocate for women's health and well-being. With years of experience working in women's health advocacy, Lila has dedicated her career to empowering women through knowledge and support.

Her journey began with a deep interest in the intricate dance of hormones within the female body and how they influence every aspect of health and daily life. Recognizing the lack of accessible, comprehensive information on the subject, Lila set out to bridge the gap between medical research and the everyday experiences of women.

Lila writes with the conviction that understanding one's body is the first step toward wellness and self-empowerment. Her work is characterized by its empathetic tone, practical advice, and unwavering commitment to debunking myths surrounding women's health.

Lila Lacy continues to be a beacon of hope and a source of cutting-edge information for women seeking to reclaim their health and harmony with their bodies. Her books not only educate but also inspire readers to make lasting changes that resonate through all facets of their lives.

When she's not writing or speaking, Lila enjoys practicing yoga, experimenting with hormone-friendly recipes, and spending time in nature.

www.ingramcontent.com/pod-product-compliance
Lightning Source LLC
Chambersburg PA
CBHW071719020426
42333CB00017B/2328